Prevention of
Venous Thrombosis and
Pulmonary Embolism

To
Ian Douglas-Wilson
Former Editor of the Lancet

Prevention of Venous Thrombosis and Pulmonary Embolism

J. G. Sharnoff
Pathologist and Director of Laboratories
The Mount Vernon Hospital
Mount Vernon, New York

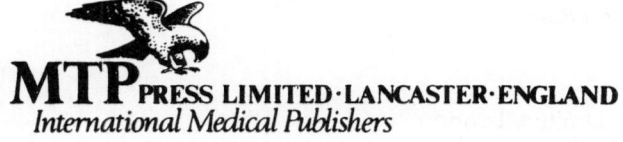

MTP **PRESS LIMITED·LANCASTER·ENGLAND**
International Medical Publishers

Published by
MTP Press Limited
Falcon House
Lancaster, England

Copyright © 1980 J. G. Sharnoff
Softcover reprint of the hardcover 1st edition 1980

First published 1980

British Library Cataloguing in Publication Data

Sharnoff, J G
    Prevention of venous thrombosis and pulmonary
    embolism.
    1. Thrombosis – Prevention   2. Veins – Diseases
    – Prevention   3. Thromboembolism – Prevention
    4. Pulmonary embolism – Prevention
    I. Title
    616.1'45'05   RC697

ISBN   978-94-009-8705-0   ISBN   978-94-009-8703-6 (eBook)
DOI: 10.1007/978-94-009-8703-6

Typeset by
Input Typesetting Limited, London

Contents

Preface

This book has been prompted by recent advances in the safe prevention of thromboembolism by subcutaneous heparin prophylaxis, in particular postoperatively. It has been correctly called by S. Sherry a major breakthrough in medicine. Although thromboembolism was first recognized by Laennec in 1819 and defined by Virchow in 1846, its development was not well understood and its prevention escaped our best efforts until now. This all-too-common, sudden, unexpected and unwanted form of morbidity and mortality, always referred to in the surgical patient as postoperative pulmonary thromboembolism, has now become the major complication of all surgery. However, it occurs with equal frequency in hospitalized non-operative patients as well, so the latter are also in need of this prophylaxis if this calamity is to be avoided. The mass of literature generated in the past few years has produced some confusion as to which of a number of methods of heparin prophylaxis gives the best results. It is the intention of this book to help clarify the situation and thereby resolve the problem by offering a procedure of subcutaneous heparin prophylaxis which is acceptable, safe and simple to administer. Recent technical advances offer the hope of attaining this goal.

Acknowledgements

I wish to acknowledge with thanks the assistance given me in preparing this book to Miss Viola Johnson, my former secretary, Mrs Mary Coan, the hospital librarian and Dr Alex Silverglade of Riker Laboratories, Inc., USA.

My special thanks to Mr A. N. Nicolaides of St Mary's Hospital, London and especially to my wife Florence for her patient and capable editing of the manuscript.

1
Epidemiology

Although Laennec first described the pulmonary infarct in 1819 and Virchow explained its development as a deep vein thrombosis and embolism to the pulmonary arteries in 1846[63], little has been accomplished since then in the prevention of this often fatal phenomenon. The reason for this is attributable to the fact that the development of thrombosis still remains partially understood. This is despite the fact that Virchow in 1856[64] described a triad for thrombosis which is still valid today; he suggested that blood stasis, vascular wall injury and alteration of the blood constituents are the main causes of thrombosis. Many complex explanations have been and are being suggested to explain the last mentioned; but so far our best efforts have failed.

With the advent of antibiotics came the conquering of most common bacterial infections and the control of some viral infections, so thromboembolism has assumed a more prominent position as a cause of morbidity and mortality. Thus, it has been estimated that more than 200 000 thromboembolisms occur in the United States annually[39,65]. In the event of death, the autopsy has disclosed an almost equal frequency of thromboembolism in both medical and surgical patients. In the latter it often occurs after operation and has therefore been referred to as postoperative pulmonary thromboembolism. However, it may also be observed with some frequency during or immediately following surgery and producing cardiopulmonary arrest and death. These deaths are to this

11

day usually attributed to anaesthesia[53,56] which has been the case since the introduction of anaesthesia with chloroform and ether. Autopsy evidence indicates that pulmonary thromboembolism is the most frequent (70%) cause of death[48]. It was deTakats[17] who described the death so aptly as 'found suddenly dead in bed'. In most instances anaesthesia is not implicated and death occurs without premonitory signs within minutes, leaving no time for embolectomy or thrombolytic therapy[11,14,23,45,59]. This makes the need for prophylactic treatment mandatory.

Fatal pulmonary thromboembolism is undoubtedly chiefly a hospital-based problem[36]. In this respect it lends further support to one of Virchow's postulates in the development of thrombosis, namely blood stasis. The hospitalized patient is greatly restricted in his movements and is often completely immobilized[48]. This induces blood stasis in the veins of the lower limbs. Although older patients are at the greatest risk, fatal pulmonary thromboembolism can occur at any age[19,31,32]. It has on occasion been reported in neonates[66], but is more frequently observed beginning with the teenage years and increasing in frequency with advancing age. Orthopaedic patients requiring surgery for hip fractures, total hip replacement and leg amputations[20,21,45-47,52] are at the greatest risk, followed by patients requiring thoracoabdominal surgery[15,26,67] and women during the early post-partum period[1,7,42]. The non-surgical patients at greatest risk in order of frequency are those with acute myocardial infarctions, congestive heart disease,[22,25,34,54,58,68] septicaemias[16], diabetes mellitus[11,36], cerebrovascular accidents, malignancy[2,8,10,40,55], obesity, and young women using oral contraceptives[3,12,13,39,44,61,62].

Fatal pulmonary thromboembolism has also been observed at post-mortem following minor surgery including dentistry. This is usually in cardiopulmonary arrest cases in association with general anaesthesia as mentioned above. Although rarely observed in non-hospitalized healthy individuals, it has been noted in individuals during prolonged airplane travel[57], television watching, and in sedentary occupations and prolonged rest periods[27,50,68]. Fatal pulmonary thromboembolism may occur in these individuals with or without the presence of lower extremity varicosities[9].

Recent reports indicate that the incidence of fatal pulmonary thromboembolism is greater in Great Britain and on the European continent than in the United States. This may not be a statistical discrepancy but a reflection on the difference in hospital care. Length of hospitalization in Great Britain is as a rule longer than in the United States. As mentioned above longer periods of immobilization are a distinct hazard[50].

Other conditions which may be associated with thromboembolism are anaemia and polycythaemia. There also appears to be a seasonal variation in the frequency of pulmonary embolism in the temperate zones, the greatest incidence being in the spring and fall[51]. It has been postulated that this seasonal difference is due to the renewed physical activity following periods of greatest inactivity during the cold of winter and the heat of summer. Tropical and subtropical areas on the other hand appear to have a lower incidence of thromboembolism. This may be explained by the lack of seasonal difference and the constant activity in all seasons[24,30,44,60]. The above is consistent with the findings in the classic study of Morris et al. on London bus employees[38]. The authors reported a higher incidence of coronary artery thrombosis in the sitting bus drivers compared with the lower incidence observed in the physically active conductors. Although these were cases of arterial thrombosis, they may well reflect the cumulative effect of coagulation factors in the immobile bus drivers and the development of hypercoagulable blood according to the third postulate of Virchow (see below).

Statistical findings tend to be either conflicting or unrevealing[14,40]. The reported incidence of pulmonary embolism as a cause of death, from the US National Center for Health Statistics, is very inaccurate. This is because of the low autopsy rate and the difficulty in differentiating pulmonary embolic death from other forms of sudden death. Thus the Vital Statistics of the United States for the year 1976[65] reported only 11 513 deaths from pulmonary embolism and infarctions, which is probably a very inaccurate figure.

The data for the incidence of pulmonary embolism according to sex reveal little difference. The US Vital Statistics indicate an almost equal distribution in males and females of approximately five deaths per 100 000, which is an unlikely figure. The crude death rate reported by Vessey and Inman[62] in England and Wales showed a lower incidence among males compared to that in females. This may be due to a greater incidence of orthopaedic problems in elderly females compared to males (five to one) and a high incidence of pulmonary emboli in pregnant females and those on the Pill. In a large sample of patients treated with anti-coagulants for venous thromboembolism Coon[14] found an equal number of males and females. In a hospital population many other illnesses must also play a role in the epidemiology of thrombo-embolism.

The effect of age on the incidence of pulmonary thromboembol-ism has long been established by reports from the United States, Britain, Australia, Germany, and Japan. These reports disclose a steady increase in the incidence of pulmonary thromboembolism with age. Dividing points according to age have been suggested; after the age of 30 years heart disease and malignancy appear to play an added role in its development. Kakkar and his colleagues[33] reported a higher frequency in postoperative patients as detected by the [^{125}I]fibrinogen uptake test in patients 60 years of age or over compared with patients 40–59 years of age. It is far less common in children. The youngest postoperative fatal thrombo-embolism observed at autopsy and reported by the author occurred in a 16-year-old black male following a right inguinal hernio-rrhaphy[48]. More recently the author also observed a fatal pulmon-ary thromboembolism in a 16-year-old black female with acute diffuse lupus erythematosus treated vigorously with corticosteroids. Emery[19] reported 25 fatal pulmonary embolisms in a sampling of 2000 autopsies in children.

Spontaneous deep vein thrombosis is not uncommon in adults but extremely rare in children, and when it does occur in the latter it is associated with injury, heart disease, malignancy, renal dis-ease, and infections.

There are a few reported instances of familial venous thrombo-embolism generally occurring when two or more members of the same family have been affected. Usually they have been reported in association with some blood defect. Most commonly it occurs in families with myelosclerosis in the presence of thrombocytosis.

There is ample confirmed evidence that oestrogens and oral contraceptives do increase the risk of venous thromboembolism developing. A recent British study[39] disclosed a seven-fold greater incidence in women on oral contraceptives than women not taking them. The dose of oestrogen has also been found to correlate with the risk of thromboembolism–the larger the dose, the greater incidence. The study of the Royal College of General Practitioners has shown that women who have been taking the Pill for 5 years or more have a five times greater mortality mainly from vascular problems.

The use of oestrogens in the treatment of heart disease, suppression of lactation and in the treatment of prostatic carcinoma is also associated with a higher incidence of thromboembolic complications. The same association has been noted with the use of diethylstilboesterol. Arterial thromboses have also been implicated in the use of oral contraceptives. As a result of the above association it has been recommended that women taking oral contraceptives and requiring surgery discontinue taking the contraceptive several weeks before operation.

Patients with certain blood types have been described as having a greater potential for developing thromboembolic complications in association with surgery[29]. The blood type most commonly associated with thromboembolism is Group A and, less commonly, Group O.

During pregnancy and the puerperium women have an increased risk of venous thrombosis and possible pulmonary embolism. It has been reported that pulmonary embolism occurs 5.5 times more frequently in pregnant than in non-pregnant women. Post-partum thrombosis has been noted to occur up to six times more frequently than ante-partum thrombosis.

Obese individuals have a greater risk of pulmonary embolism than the non-obese. This was well documented by the studies of Kakkar and his colleagues[33] and by Nicolaides and Irving[40]. These studies employed the $[^{125}I]$fibrinogen scanning technique to determine the increased frequency of deep vein thrombosis in obese individuals.

The relative frequency of deep vein thrombosis and pulmonary embolism in hospitalized patients with heart disease as demonstrated at autopsy is well documented. Coon has reported[14] that pulmonary embolism is 3½ times as frequent in patients over the age of 30 years with heart disease than those of the same age without heart disease. Coon[14] has also reported that all types of heart disease, excluding hypertensive congenital heart disease, have a significantly increased risk of pulmonary embolism. The likelihood of embolism is even greater in patients with atrial fibrillation and in congestive heart disease. Patients with acute myocardial infarction also have a great risk of developing deep vein thrombosis and fatal pulmonary thromboembolism, a fact confirmed from autopsy findings in 25% of cases. Deep vein thrombosis has been shown to occur in acute myocardial infarction in 30–40% of patients as determined by the [125I]fibrinogen uptake in the leg veins by Handley, Emerson and Fleming[25]. It has been determined that more than one-half of these thrombi develop within 72 hours of the acute myocardial infarction. Advanced age and varicose veins increase the risk in these patients.

The association of venous thrombosis with cancer has long been known. Migratory superficial venous thrombosis has been observed frequently and particularly with carcinoma of the pancreas[55]. It has also been reported in patients with carcinoma of the lung[10] and stomach. An increased risk of venous thrombosis and embolism is also associated with many other types of malignancy[2]. There is an overall two- to three-fold increase in thromboembolism in all patients with cancer. Other reports indicate that over 40% of patients with cancer develop evidence of deep vein thrombosis, and that there is a three-fold increase in the risk of postoperative thrombosis in all patients with malignancy. There have been many studies made in an attempt to explain this association with malignancy including studies on clotting factors, blood viscosity and platelets[8] but so far there have been no clear-cut results. It is more likely that other factors such as age and prolonged bed rest following surgery are more significant in the development of venous thromboembolism.

A past history of deep vein thrombosis poses another risk. This must be considered an added risk when operation is contemplated. This has been well documented in studies by Barker et al.[4] and by Nicolaides and Irving[40]; the latter reported a frequency of 61% in deep vein thrombosis.

Varicose veins have long been cited as an added risk in surgical patients. Barker et al.[4] reported that in patients undergoing abdominal hysterectomy there was a three-fold increase in the frequency of thromboembolic disease if there was a history of peripheral vein disease. Nicolaides and Irving[40] reported a two-fold increase in risk in postoperative patients if varicose veins were present.

The correlation between trauma and burns and the development of venous thrombosis has also been well documented by Sevitt and Gallagher[47]. Most of the deep vein thromboses lack clinical signs, the incidence decreasing with distance from the site of injury. Thus, head injuries have the lowest incidence, chest injuries and burns have a higher incidence, and the highest (60%) occurs in patients with pelvic and femoral fractures[46,52] and, as stated above, bed rest appears to play an important role here.

Deep vein thrombosis has always been a complication of acute infectious disease, especially bloodstream infections. This is especially true of Gram-negative sepsis. However, other organisms such as the pneumococci, meningococci, and streptococci in the blood have also been implicated as causing disseminated intravascular coagulation (DIC). Bindschadler and Bennett[6] have also reported infusion thrombophlebitis as a frequent complication of fungal infections. They recommend adding 1000 units of heparin per 500 ml dextrose to the infusion bottle.

Most attention has been paid to patients with hip fractures. Fitts et al.[21] reported a 38% incidence of fatal pulmonary thromboembolism observed at autopsy in all deaths following hip fractures. Others have reported a higher incidence (50% and 86%) of deep vein thrombosis following hip fractures[47,52]. The overall incidence of postoperative fatalities for non-anticoagulated hip fractures has been reported by the author and his colleagues as 3.5%[52] in a review of 403 cases. It was indicated that trauma *per se* to the injured limb is not the decisive factor in the development of deep vein thrombosis since both limbs are usually affected with vein thrombi. It would appear that the immobilization following injury is an additional decisive factor. Direct trauma to the veins and the resultant development of thrombosis at the site of injury can be explained without difficulty.

The long list of risk factors detailed here implies that the cause of thrombosis is still not completely understood. It also leads to confusion in attempting to determine which individual should receive prophylactic treatment for deep vein thrombosis. Two factors appear to run through the entire list of risks: these are venous stasis and hypercoagulability, with thrombosis forming where stasis is most likely to be present, namely in the leg veins. This may well explain why thromboembolism is a common problem of the hospitalized and surgical patient. As will be explained below the stress of surgery induces the development of hypercoagulable blood which produces thrombosis in areas of stasis such as the veins of limbs with limited activity or immobilization.

It would appear that prophylaxis is essential for the above individuals if thromboembolism is to be avoided. If thrombosis and embolism occur at any age, with the simplest procedures and, as often happens, in so-called non-risk patients, then all operative and hospitalized patients deserve a safe, effective, easily monitored means of prevention. This is especially true in view of the fact that there is no reliable test capable of predicting which patients are at risk. As will be indicated in later chapters the so-called 'screening' tests for the detection of deep vein thrombosis are not reliable and often become positive too late (that is after the formation of thrombi).

References

1. Aaro, L. A. and Juergens, J. L. (1974). Thrombophlebitis and pulmonary embolism as complications of pregnancy. *Med. Clin. N. Am.*, **58**, 829
2. Amundsen, M. A., Spittel, J. A. Jr., Thompson, J. H. Jr. and Owen, C. A. Jr. (1963). Hypercoagulability associated with malignant disease and with the postoperative state. *Ann. Intern. Med.*, **56**, 608
3. Badaracco, M. A. and Vessey, M. P. (1974). Recurrence of venous thromboembolic disease and use of oral contraceptives. *Br. Med. J.*, **1**, 215
4. Barker, N. W., Nygaard, K. K., Walters, W. and Priestley, J. T. (1941). A statistical study of postoperative venous thrombosis and pulmonary embolism – predisposing factors. *Mayo Clin. Proc.*, **16**, 1
5. Bennett, N. B., Ogston, C. W., McAndrew, G. W. and Ogston, D. (1966). Studies on the fibrinolytic enzyme system in obesity. *J. Clin. Pathol.*, **19**, 241
6. Bindschadler, D.D. and Bennett, J. E. (1969). A pharmocologic guide to the clinical use of Amphotericin B. *J. Infect. Dis.*, **120**, 427
7. Bonnar, J., McNicol, G. P. and Douglas, A. S. (1970). Coagulation and fibrinolytic mechanisms during and after normal childbirth. *Br. Med. J.*, **2**, 200
8. Brugarolas, A., Mink, I. B., Elias, E. G. and Mittelman, A. (1973). Correlation of hyperfibrinogenemia with thromboembolism in patients with cancer. *Surg. Gynecol. Obstet.*, **136**, 75
9. Burkitt, D. P. (1972). Varicose veins, deep vein thrombosis and haemorrhoids: epidemiology and suggested aetiology. *Br. Med. J.*, **2**, 556
10. Byrd, R. E., Divertie, M. B. and Spittel, J. A. Jr. (1967). Bronchogenic carcinoma and thromboembolic disease. *J. Am. Med. Assoc.*, **202**, 219
11. Carlotti, J., Hardy, I. B. Jr., Linton, R. R. and White, P. D. (1947). Pulmonary embolism in medical patients. *Am. Heart J.*, **33**, 737
12. Carvalho, A. C. A., Vaillancourt, R. A., Cabral, R. B., Lees, R. S. and Colman, R. W. (1977). Coagulation abnormalities in women taking oral contraceptives. *J. Am. Med. Assoc.*, **237**, 875
13. Caspary, E. A. and Peperdy, M. (1965). Oral contraception and blood platelet adhesiveness. *Lancet*, **1**, 1142

14. Coon, W. W. (1976). Epidemiology of venous thromboembolism. *Ann. Surg.*, **186**, 149

15. Coon, W. W. (1976). Risk factors in pulmonary embolism. *Surg. Gynecol. Obstet.*, **143**, 385

16. Corrigan, J. J. Jr. (1977). Heparin therapy in bacterial septicemia. *J. Pediatr.*, **91**, 65

17. deTakats, G. (1950). Anticoagulation in surgery. *J. Am. Med. Assoc.*, **142**, 527

18. Donaldson, G. A., Williams, C., Scannell, J. G. and Shaw, R. S. (1950). A reappraisal of the application of the Trendelenburg operation to massive fatal embolism. *N. Engl. J. Med.*, **268**, 171

19. Emery, J. L. (1962). Pulmonary embolism in children. *Arch. Dis. Child.*, **37**, 591

20. Fisher, W., Michele, A. and McCann, W. (1963). Thrombophlebitis and pulmonary infarction associated with fractured hip. *Clin. Res.*, **11**, 407

21. Fitts, W. T. Jr., Lehr, H. B., Bittner, R. L. and Spelman, J. W. (1964). An analysis of 950 fatal injuries. *Surgery*, **56**, 663

22. Gore, I., Hirst, A. E. and Taraka, K. (1964). Myocardial infarction and thromboembolism. *Arch. Intern. Med.*, **113**, 323

23. Gorham, L. W. (1961). A study of pulmonary embolism. *Arch. Intern. Med.*, **108**, 8

24. Halse, T. Jr. and Quernet, G. (1948). Zur Frage der klimatischen Einflusse in die Thrombogenese. *Beitr. Klin. Chir.*, **177**, 287

25. Handley, A. J., Emerson, P. A. and Fleming, P. R. (1972). Heparin in the prevention of deep vein thrombosis after myocardial infarction. *Br. Med. J.*, **2**, 436

26. Hirsh, J. (1975). Venous thromboembolism diagnosis, treatment and prevention. *Hosp. Pract.*, **10**, 53

27. Homans, J. (1954). Thrombosis of the deep leg veins due to prolonged sitting. *N. Engl. J. Med.*, **250**, 148

28. Inman, W.H.W. and Vessey, M. P. (1968). Investigation of deaths from pulmonary coronary and cerebral thrombosis and embolism in women of child-bearing age. *Br. Med. J.*, **2**, 193

29. Jick, H., Slone, D., Westerholm, B., Inman, W.H.W., Vessey, M.P., Shapiro, S., Lewis, G. P. and Worcester, J. (1969). Venous thromboembolic disease and ABO blood type. A cooperative study. *Lancet*, **1**, 539

30. Joffe, S. W. (1974). Racial incidence of postoperative deep vein thrombosis in South Africa. *Br. J. Surg.*, **61**, 982

31. Joffe, S. (1975). Postoperative deep vein thrombosis in children. *J. Pediatr. Surg.*, **10**, 539

32. Jones, D. R. and MacIntyre, I. M. (1975). Venous thromboembolism in infancy and childhood. *Arch. Dis. Child.*, **50**, 153

33. Kakkar, V. V., Nicolaides, A. N., Renney, J. T. G., Friend, J. R. and Clarke, M. B. (1970). [125]I labelled fibrinogen test adapted for routine screening for deep vein thrombosis. *Lancet*, **1**, 540

34. Mauer, B. J., Wray, R. and Schillingford, J. P. (1971). Frequency of deep venous thrombosis after myocardial infarction. *Lancet*, **2**, 1385

35. McCartney, J. S. (1934). Pulmonary embolism following trauma. *Am. J. Pathol.*, **10**, 209

36. Morrell, M. T. and Dunnill, M. S. (1968). The post mortem incidence of pulmonary embolism in a hospital population. *Br. J. Surg.*, **55**, 347

37. Morrell, M. T. (1976). Acute illness – an important cause of venous thrombosis and pulmonary embolism. *Br. J. Surg.*, **63**, 162

38. Morris, J. N., Heady, J., Raffle, P. A., Roberts, O. G. and Parks, R. W. (1953). Coronary heart disease and physical activity of work. *Lancet*, **2**, 1053

39. Mortality among oral contraceptive users (1977). Royal College of General Practitioners Oral Contraceptive Study. *Lancet*, **2**, 727

40. Nicolaides, A. N. and Irving, D. (1975). Clinical factors and the risk of deep venous thrombosis. In A. N. Nicolaides (ed.). *Thromboembolism* (Lancaster: MTP Press)

41. Ochsner, A. (1954). Advances in surgery of the colon. *Am. J. Surg.*, **88**, 807

42. Ramsay, D. M. (1975). Thromboembolism in pregnancy. *Obstet. Gynecol.*, **45**, 129

43. Rossman, I. (1974). True incidence of pulmonary embolization and vital statistics. *J. Am. Med. Assoc.*, **230**, 1677

44. Sandritter, W. and Felix, H. (1967). Geographical pathology of fatal lung embolism. *Pathol. Microbiol.*, **30**, 742

45. Sevitt, S. (1968). Fatal road accident injuries, complications and causes of death in 250 subjects. *Br. J. Surg.*, **55**, 481

46. Sevitt, S. (1962). Venous thrombosis and pulmonary embolism, their prevention by oral anticoagulants. *Am. J. Med.*, **33**, 703

47. Sevitt, S. and Gallagher, N. (1961). Venous thrombosis and pulmonary embolism. A clinicopathological study in injured and burned patients. *Br. J. Surg.*, **48**, 475

48. Sharnoff, J. G. (1966). Post mortem findings in 25 cases of sudden heart arrest in the perioperative period. *Lancet*, **2**, 876

49. Sharnoff, J. G. (1969). Prevention of sudden cardio-pulmonary arrest in the perioperative period with prophylactic heparin. *Lancet*, **2**, 292

50. Sharnoff, J. G. and Rosenberg, M. (1964). Effects of age and immobilization on the incidence of postoperative thromboembolism. *Lancet*, **1**, 845

51. Sharnoff, J. G., Rosenberg, M. and Mistica, B. A. (1963). Seasonal variation in fatal thromboembolism and its high incidence in the surgical patient. *Surg. Gynecol. Obstet.*, **116**, 11

52. Sharnoff, J. G., Rosen, R. L., Sadler, A. H. and Ibarra-Isunza, G. C. (1976). Prevention of fatal pulmonary thromboembolism by heparin prophylaxis after surgery for hip fractures. *J. Bone Jt. Surg.*, **58–A**, 913

53. Sibson, H. (1848). Chloroform anaesthesia as a cause of death. *Lond. Med. Gaz.*, **42**, 108

54. Simmons, A. V., Sheppard, M. A. and Cox, A. F. (1973). Deep venous thrombosis after myocardial infarction. *Br. Heart J.*, **35**, 623

55. Sproul, E. E. (1938). Carcinoma and venous thrombosis: frequency of association of carcinoma in body or tail of pancreas with multiple venous thrombosis. *Am. J. Cancer*, **34**, 566

56. Stephenson, H. E. Jr., Reid, C. L. and Hinton, W. J. (1953). Some common denominators in 1200 cases of cardiac arrest. *Ann. Surg.*, **137**, 731

57. Symington, I. S. and Stack, B. H. R. (1977). Pulmonary thromboembolism after travel. *Br. J. Dis. Chest*, **71**, 138
58. Thomas, W. A., Davies, J. N. P., O'Neal, R. M. and Dimakalangan, A. A. (1960). Incidence of myocardial infarction correlated with venous and pulmonary thrombosis and embolism: a geographic study based on autopsies in Uganda, East Africa and St Louis, USA. *Am. J. Cardiol.*, **5**, 41
59. Towbin, A. (1954). Pulmonary embolism: incidence and significance. *J. Am. Med. Assoc.*, **156**, 209
60. Trousseau, A. (1865). Phlegmasie alba dolens. Clinique Medicale de L'Hotel-Dieu de Paris Ballière, Paris, p. 94
61. Vessey, M. P. and Mann, J. I. (1978). Female sex hormones and thrombosis: epidemiological aspects. *Br. Med. Bull.*, **34**, 157
62. Vessey, M P. and Inman, W. H. W. (1973). Speculations about mortality trends from venous thromboembolic disease in England and Wales and their relation to the pattern of oral contraceptive usage. *Br. J. Obstet. Gynaecol.*, **80**, 562
63. Virchow, R. (1846). Die verstopfung der Lungen arterie und ihre Folgen. *Beitr. Exp. Pathol. Physiol.*, **2**, 1
64. Virchow, R. (1856). *Gesammelte Abhandlungen zur Wissenschaftlichen Medezin.* (Frankfurt-am-Main: von Meidinger Sohn)
65. Vital Statistics of the United States, Vol. 11, Mortality Part A for 1976
66. Wesley, J. R., Keens, T. G., Miller, S. W. and Platzker, C. G. (1978). Pulmonary embolism in the neonate: occurrence during the course of total parenteral nutrition. *J. Pediatr.*, **93**, 113
67. Wessler, S. (1977). The anticoagulant dilemma: a prescription for its resolution. *Am. J. Med. Sci.*, **274**, 106
68. White, P. D. (1940). Pulmonary embolism and heart disease: a review of twenty years of personal experience. *Am. J. Med. Sci.*, **200**, 577

2

Pathology of Thrombi

Coagulation of the blood is normally essential to arrest bleeding. However, blood coagulation within the circulatory system is abnormal and the haemostatic plug which forms from the elements of the flowing blood is referred to as a thrombus. A thrombus may also form as a reparative process when there is a break in a vessel wall. If too great a reaction causes a thrombus large enough to obstruct the flow of blood this is a pathological state. Circulating blood contains all the elements necessary to form a solid coagulum at the site of injury to the vessel wall. A break in the wall causing haemorrhage prompts an immediate reaction. Platelets separate from the extravasating blood, adhere to each other and to the edges of the break to initiate the haemostatic plug. Leukocytes and red blood cells may be incorporated in the plug. Fibrin then covers the platelet plug producing a more stable mass. Circumstances such as the rate of blood flow and the hypercoagulable state of the blood[5,10] will then determine whether the plug will become abnormal as an obstructing thrombus.

All thrombi have a distinctive structure histologically due to the selective accumulation of platelets and leukocytes in flowing blood, held together by fibrin[5,7].

Thrombi are sometimes simple in structure, composed chiefly of one element or a mixture of several elements. The *simple thrombi* are those composed of platelets, fibrin or erythrocytes; they are

23

rarely seen in the pure form. *Platelet thrombi* may have small amounts of fibrin and *fibrin thrombi* may have a few platelets[6].

Platelet thrombi are usually seen in small blood vessels, chiefly arteries or on heart leaflets. They are composed of closely packed aggregates of platelets and fibrin is usually deposited on their surface[11].

Fibrin thrombi have a distinctive appearance differing from other thrombi. They are composed chiefly of closely packed strands of fibrin with a few non-aggregated entrapped platelets. They are usually noted in small vessels, especially capillaries.

Red cell thrombi are masses of aggregated erythrocytes. They are observed as irregularly shaped masses and rouleaux aggregates in the smaller blood vessels such as arterioles, capillaries and venules. They can be observed experimentally but are not generally seen in tissues[10].

The *mixed thrombi* are the most common. They are composed of platelets, leukocytes and fibrin and may reach any size. They form in arteries, veins and the heart. The proportion of their various elements may differ, but usually the erythrocytes make up the bulk of the mass. Their basic structure is the same. Platelet aggregates are seen surrounded by fibrin and leukocytes in characteristic arrangement. Fibrin may be seen between the platelets and on the free surfaces of the platelet aggregates with their fine strands incorporating the leukocytes on the fringe of the aggregates[5].

There are two ways in which thrombi may begin. When they originate on an injured vessel wall they are referred to as *in situ* thrombi. They may also originate in the bloodstream and are then called intravascular thrombi or emboli. As unattached thrombi they pose the danger of embolization. *In situ* thrombi form on areas of diseased vessel wall caused by arteriosclerosis or injury. The platelets are first seen to adhere to the sites of disease or injury. Slowing of the bloodstream and eddying, as in dilated areas, are important factors contributing to this phenomenon. Fibrin appears to form later to incorporate the mass of platelets. It is generally accepted that thrombi form at sites where the endothelium is lost, but not where it is intact[3]. The platelets stick together by cohesion and do not fuse together, apparently adhering to the collagen fibres of the subendothelial layer; they may swell and change their shape and this aids in their aggregation[20].

The appearance of fibrin which follows the aggregation of platelets is probably derived from released platelet fibrinogen. By incorporating the platelet aggregates it limits the shape of the thrombus; and by their adhesion platelets contribute to thrombin generation which also alters the platelet aggregates. As a thrombus continues to develop, fibrin enmeshes the leukocytes and erythrocytes in the mass. It appears that there is a selectivity in the process of entrapping the leukocytes and red cells in the fibrin. The granulocytes and monocytes are entrapped but not the lymphocytes. The former are usually found on the periphery and the monocytes appear to act by phagocytosis in the resolution of thrombotic material[5,8,21].

Intravascular thrombi which form entirely within the bloodstream are produced by thrombogenic stimuli introduced or generated within the blood. They are usually mixed platelet fibrin thrombi which lodge eventually in smaller blood vessels where they may cause ischaemic necrosis. Experimentally, these thrombi may be produced by the injection of procoagulant substances, antigen–antibody complexes, adenosine diphosphates, fatty acids and thrombin. Foreign substances and micro-organisms when introduced into the blood may also produce these thrombi. The introduction of such substances as thromboplastin and Russel's viper venom rapidly produces thrombin which induces the formation of platelet–fibrin thrombi[16]. Gram-negative bacterial endotoxins introduced into the bloodstream experimentally are also capable of producing intravascular thrombi. These produce ischaemic necrosis and haemorrhage as in the Shwartzman reaction. Lee[13] in a classic experiment demonstrated that the slow infusion of dilute thrombin was capable of producing the Shwartzman phenomenon. This showed conclusively that endotoxins alone were not the only means of producing intravascular thrombi, but that perhaps the endotoxins generate thrombin in the bloodstream activating the coagulation system. Aggregated platelets are known to release thrombin and are therefore another local means of activating the coagulation system.

In man, the development of emboli from intravascular mixed

thrombi is a significant means of promoting disease. This is exemplified by bacterial and viral infections in which microembolic thrombosis produces ischaemic and haemorrhagic lesions[14,15]. Meningococcaemia in acute form produces the Shwartzman phenomenon and is also capable of producing the Waterhouse–Friedrichsen syndrome as seen in the bilateral haemorrhagic infarction of the adrenal glands. The Shwartzman reaction may also be noted in abruptio placenta and septic abortion. Intravascular embolic thrombi can also develop in chronic disease such as malignancy, and the association with carcinoma of the pancreas has already been mentioned in the previous chapter.

The differentiation between *in situ* and embolic thrombi is not always possible. For example, the thrombotic phenomena noted in thrombotic thrombocytopenic purpura have not been clearly explained as to whether they are due to vascular injury or are, as is more likely, of embolic nature. The depletion of blood factors especially the thrombocytopenia which accompanies it, places this condition in the category of consumption coagulopathy or disseminated intravascular coagulation. Acute peptic stress ulcers with their exsanguinating haemorrhages and possible bowel perforations may be another example of *in situ* or embolic thrombosis. The thrombosed vessels which are observed in the submucosa of these ulcers are the cause of the ischaemic necrosis in the mucosa and the ulcerations which follow lead to massive haemorrhages, perforation of the bowel resulting in acute diffuse peritonitis[17].

Deep vein thromboses which develop in the leg veins are caused by several factors. These are increased coagulable properties of the blood, platelet reaction and slowing of blood flow. The release reaction of platelets, the slowing of the blood and its eddying in the valve pockets of the leg veins often lead to the initiation of thrombi at these sites[17]; with their formation there is further retardation of blood flow leading to propagation of the thrombus in both directions but chiefly in the direction of blood flow. These are the 'red thrombi' of the deep leg veins which may be loosely attached and easily freed to cause emboli to the pulmonary arteries, producing sudden shock and possibly death.

The slowing of venous blood flow in association with the release of thrombogenic substances would appear to be an essential component in the production of deep vein thrombosis. The most important thrombogenic substance released from platelets is thrombin. This combination of factors which causes thrombosis occurs most frequently in patients with congestive heart failure, after major thoracoabdominal surgery in the perioperative period and especially in immobilized elderly patients suffering hip fractures who have the highest risk[9,19]. Further examples of disturbance in blood flow leading to thrombosis are often noted in patients with cardiac arrythmias. The auricular appendages frequently develop thrombi, especially between the trabecular muscles. Acute myocardial infarction with its disturbed myocardial pulsations and endocardial reactions are a common site of thrombus formation. Also, healed myocardial infarcts with aneurysm formation cause turbulence and slowed blood flow leading to laminated thrombus formation.

Increased blood viscosity as in polycythaemia vera is also believed to predispose to thrombus formation. This is less likely in the larger blood vessels, despite the higher concentration of red blood cells, than in the smaller veins and arteries. The accompanying thrombocytosis in this disease may also play a significant role.

The concept of blood hypercoagulability has always been elusive. Recently it has been considered to be a latent thrombotic state of the blood with all normal coagulation factors present wherein the capacity of an increased production of thrombin exists. A decrease in certain coagulation factors, as in haemorrhagic diseases, does not lead to a thrombotic state, nor is an increase in these factors usually associated with thrombosis. However, reports appearing in the literature would indicate that in some instances venous thromboembolism has been connected with increased levels of factors V and VIII and also with the presence of abnormal fibrinogen. Conversely, there are reports indicating that thrombosis is associated with decreased levels of antithrombin III, a natural anticoagulant which inhibits the activation of the procoagulants factor X and thrombin[21].

Other reports indicate that thrombosis in arterial disease may be associated with platelet function and altered lipids. Hyper-

27

coagulability has been reported with increased platelet phospholipids in patients with coronary artery disease, diabetes mellitus and familial hyperlipoproteinaemia. A sudden increase in plasma-free fatty acids has also been implicated in hypercoagulation as a result of stress and the release of catecholamines.

A possible external source of platelet microemboli may be introduced during massive blood transfusions. As with other microthromboemboli produced *in vivo* they are capable of causing symptoms by cerebral and pulmonary embolization. This has led to a search for blood filters for use in transfusions to prevent such complications[12].

References

1. Allison, P. R., Dunnill, M. S. and Marshall, R. (1960). Pulmonary embolism. *Thorax*, **15**, 273
2. Aschoff, L. (1913). Thrombosis. *Arch. Intern. Med.*, **12**, 503
3. Ashford, T. P. and Freiman, D. G. (1967). The role of the endothelium in the initial phases of thrombosis. *Am. J. Pathol.*, **50**, 257
4. Bizzozero, J. (1882). Über einem neuen formbestandtheil des Blutes und dessen Rolle bei der Thrombose und Blutgerinnung. *Virchows Arch. Pathol. Anat. Physiol.*, **90**, 261
5. Chandler, A. B. (1969). The anatomy of a thrombus. In Sherry, S., Brinkhous, K.M., Genton, E. and Stengle, J. M. (eds.). *Thrombosis*, p. 279. (Washington: National Academy of Sciences)
6. Chandler, A. B. (1973). The platelet in thrombus formation. In Brinkhous, K. M., Sherman, R. W. and Mostofi, F. K. (eds.). *The Platelet*, p. 183. (Baltimore: Williams and Wilkins Co.)
7. Eberth, J. D. and Schimmelbusch, C. (1886). Experimentelle untersuchungen über thrombose. *Virchows Arch. Pathol. Anat. Physiol.*, **103**, 39
8. Evans, G. and Mustard, J. F. (1968). Platelet–surface reaction and thrombosis. *Surgery*, **64**, 273
9. Field, E. S., Nicolaides, A. N., Kakkar, V. V. and Crellin, R. Q. (1972). Deep-vein thrombosis in patients with fractures of femoral neck. *Br. J. Surg.*, **59**, 377
10. French, J. E. (1965). The structure of natural and experimental thrombi. *Ann. R. Coll. Surg.*, **36**, 191
11. French, J. E., MacFarlane, R. G. and Sanders, A. G. (1964). The structure of haemostatic plugs and experimental thrombi in small arteries. *Br. J. Exp. Pathol.*, **45**, 467
12. Kennedy, P. S., Solis, R. T., Scott, M. A. and Wilson, R. K. (1977). An evaluation of several blood transfusion filters. *Transfusion*, **17**, 563
13. Lee, R. E. (1955). Anatomical and physiological aspects of the capillary bed in the bulbar conjunctiva of man in health and disease. *Angiology*, **6**, 369

14. Margaretten, W. (1967). Local tissue damage in disseminated intravascular clotting. *Am. J. Cardiol.*, **20**, 185
15. McKay, D. G. (1969). Progress in disseminated intravascular coagulation. *Calif. Med.*, **111**, 186
16. Mustard, J. F., Rowsell, H. C. and Murphy, E. A. (1964). Thrombosis. *Am. J. Med. Sci.*, **248**, 469
17. Nicolaides, A. N., Kakkar, V. V. and Renney, J. T. (1971). Soleal sinuses and stasis. *Br. J. Surg.*, **58**, 307
18. Paterson, J. C. (1969). The pathology of venous thrombi. In Sherry, S., Brinkhous, K.M., Genton, E. and Stengle, J.M. (eds.). *Thrombosis*, p. 321. (Washington: National Academy of Sciences)
19. Sevitt, S. and Gallagher, N. G. (1961). Venous thrombosis and pulmonary embolism. *Br. J. Surg.*, **48**, 475
20. Ts'ao, C. H. and Glagov, S. (1970). Platelet adhesion to subendothelial components in experimental aortic injury. *Br. J. Exp. Pathol.*, **51**, 423
21. Walsh, P. N. and Biggs, R. (1972). The role of platelets in intrinsic factor Xa formation. *Br. J. Haematol.*, **22**, 743

3

Pathology of Venous Thrombosis and Pulmonary Thromboembolism

Since the days of Rokitansky and Virchow, the post-mortem examination still remains the most accurate means of determining the presence of pulmonary thromboembolism. It has been estimated[1,10,19,20] that pulmonary thromboembolism may well be the most common cause of death in the hospitalized patient. Reichel[16] indicated that careful post-mortem examination has revealed a 64% incidence of pulmonary thromboembolism in these patients. The differences in the reported incidence depends on the thoroughness with which the pulmonary arteries are examined at the autopsy table and the lung sections under the microscope. Thromboemboli can vary greatly in size. The largest have the calibre of the deep veins of the lower extremities and the pelvis, and are easily recognized; they are often found coiled in the right heart ventricle or impacted in the main stem of the pulmonary artery. Further smaller thromboemboli are often discovered in the secondary branches of the right and left pulmonary artery and have the calibre of the deeper smaller leg veins or the tributaries of the pelvic veins. Still smaller emboli may be noted by carefully examining the cut surfaces of the lungs where they can be seen protruding as firm thrombotic masses from the smaller branches of the pulmonary arteries. The smallest emboli are the micro-thromboemboli which can only be discovered by light microscopy; they are usually noted in all lung samples, and are often multiple in each section and generally many times larger than fat emboli.

There is considerable difference of opinion as to whether all of the above may explain a death in any given case. Most observers agree that the largest emboli are a competent cause of death. Yet on rare occasions large thromboemboli can be found partly organized and adherent to the intimal surfaces of the branches of the main stem pulmonary arteries indicating an earlier embolization which the patient survived. As for the smaller emboli, it appears that many may not cause death. The decision as to cause of death may well depend on clinical evidence such as the terminal condition of the patient and the manner in which death occurred. In the latter case, sudden shock and death appears to be the usual manner of death by emboli. It was this which prompted deTakats[7] to describe it as 'found suddenly dead in bed'. The condition of the patient is also of vital importance in the overall evaluation of the cause of death. Patients with heart disease, malignancy, septicaemia or other debilitating illnesses may also succumb more readily to smaller thromboemboli. Most controversial is the question of microthromboemboli, which may often precede the final large thromboembolism that caused death. On investigation there is often clinical evidence of an earlier episode of shock which the patient survived. On occasions, microthromboembolism may be found where none of the above circumstances are present. These usually occur with a patient under anaesthesia and shock cannot be readily observed until vital signs suddenly cease and the patient may or may not be resuscitated. There is sufficient experimental evidence to support the concept that microthromboemboli may be a competent cause of death. In earlier studies Wright[24] had shown that in dogs either large or very small inert masses introduced intravenously were capable of causing shock and often death. In addition, it is generally accepted that finding pulmonary fat emboli in fracture cases, which are also of microscopic size, may be designated as a cause of death. These often appear as bone marrow particles in the smallest segments of the pulmonary arteries, following hip fractures or unsuccessful attempts at cardiac resuscitation.

As mentioned above, the source of thromboemboli is generally accepted as the deep veins of the lower extremities or pelvis in over

90% of cases. According to Sevitt[18] and others[13,15] the most common sites of origin are the junctions of the deep and superficial veins of the thigh and the valve pockets of the larger deep veins. It is believed that the eddying of blood in the valve sinuses plays an important role in the origin of these thrombi.

The understanding of the pathogenesis of these thrombi, their formation and eventual embolization is vital to the development of methods of prevention. It is here that Virchow's triad may still be applied. Sevitt[18] and others hold the opinion that blood stasis plays an important role. Others[2,21] hold that trauma to the vessel wall and injury to the intima exposes collagen which initiates the formation of thrombi. In recent years the third postulate of Virchow has gained more supportive evidence; this refers to the alterations in the blood itself, designated as blood hypercoagulability. The latter is attributed to the blood platelets whose role is still not clearly defined.

It may well be that all three factors play an important role in the formation of thrombi. Vessel wall trauma may well lead to an adherent thrombus induced by an inflammatory process. The results may be a thrombophlebitis, and as an adherent clot it is least likely to embolize. Blood stasis and hypercoagulability are more likely to cause bland thrombi or phlebothrombosis. These are not adherent to the vessel wall, clinically not readily detectable and more likely to become released and terminate as lethal pulmonary emboli. To prevent this from occurring prophylaxis is required; the recent flood of reports indicate that subcutaneous heparin prophylaxis has significantly accomplished this and is now the method against which all other forms of prophylaxis should be compared. To quote a recent *Lancet* editorial, 'Heparin is still the most versatile and useful drug for prophylaxis and treatment of venous thromboembolism'. The editorial goes on to say that the prime action of heparin is to enhance the rate at which antithrombin III and α_2-globulin proteinase inhibitors neutralize certain important clotting enzymes. Heparin in combination with the above, it is theorized, neutralizes activated factor Xa and thrombin, thus preventing fibrin formation and thrombosis. It is believed that cessation of heparin therapy in patients with phlebothrombosis halts the antithrombin III neutralizing activity and leads to renewed intraluminal clotting or thrombosis, but the evidence for this is scanty. Nevertheless, intravenous heparin may be limited and unnecessary. It is recommended that subcutaneous heparin or warfarin be used in order to avoid the all too common complication of haemorrhage with intravenous heparin.

What is the natural outcome of pulmonary embolism? According to the excellent study of Dalen and Alpert[4], 16% of patients with massive pulmonary thromboembolism die before therapy can be initiated. The prognosis of the remaining 84% is generally good if no further episodes occur. Effective therapy may accomplish this by preventing further deep vein thrombosis, although if residual deep vein thrombosis is already present another and perhaps fatal episode may occur. In the hospitalized patient the cause of death in the presence of thromboembolism should be evaluated in the context of any other disease. It would appear that any embolus may be the immediate terminating event.

For the patients who survive the immediate embolic event the prognosis is reasonably good if they overcome shock and their vascular obstruction begins to clear; the latter is more likely to be due to the change in the position of the thrombus rather than to fibrinolysis which sets in early, but slowly. This has been shown in laboratory animals by Dalen, Mathur and Evans[5], who observed a change in the lung vessel obstructive phenomena using radio-opaque clots injected in the veins of dogs. It is also possible that the obstructing emboli may fragment and thereby alter and relieve the site of obstruction, thus allowing restoration of blood flow. According to Dalen, Mathur and Evans, pulmonary vascular obstruction may occur within 1–2 hours of embolism in dogs[5].

In the surviving patient, there are other changes in the embolus which can alter vascular obstruction. It has been documented[9] that a 50% reduction in the size of the embolus may be noted within 3 hours. The embolus may adhere to the pulmonary artery wall and undergo organization which will cause further shrinking of the embolus leading to an even greater decrease in the size of the embolic mass[3]. As assessed by autopsy studies this is a relatively slow process. Heparinization may also lead to a decrease in the size of the embolus by preventing propagation of the thrombotic mass which develops by accretion of fibrin and formed blood elements. The urokinase pulmonary embolism trial[25] demonstrated by lung scan and angiograms that only a slight reduction in the size of the acute thromboembolism occurred within 24 hours. This was also observed by Dalen *et al.*[3] using angiograms to occur 1–3 days after documentation of the embolic episode.

The rate of resolution of the embolism may vary depending on the area of pulmonary obstruction. Tow and Wagner[22] using lung scans observed the earliest improvement at 6 days and complete recovery at 8 days. Complete resolution at 60 days was also noted[17] in large areas of lung involvement.

The haemodynamic effects of pulmonary embolism, namely pulmonary hypertension and right ventricular enlargement and failure, resolve with resolution of the emboli. However, with repeated embolic episodes and failure of early resolution, the pulmonary hypertension and right ventricular enlargement may persist.

Another effect of pulmonary embolism is the possibility of infarction. This is not commonly seen in normal lungs, perhaps because of the double blood supply. In the event of embolism infarction is usually observed in compromised lungs. This is most often seen in patients with cardiac failure and pulmonary congestion, in pulmonary disease or in patients with prolonged inactivity[11,14]. Radiologically the infarct appears as a parenchymal density extending to the periphery[8]. However, not all infarcts extend to the pleural surface; it has been shown that infarcts may also have a lobular configuration conforming to the pulmonary lobules[12]. This may explain the variety of configurations seen radiologically in the presence of small infarcts. Larger infarcts can be readily recognized by their wedge shape involving a number of lobules and extending to the pleura. They are large areas of pulmonary tissue with intra-alveolar fibrin deposition and interstitial, periarterial and intra-alveolar haemorrhage. The pulmonary tissue undergoes necrosis which explains the density seen on plain X-ray film.

The haemorrhages that occur in pulmonary infarcts are still not adequately explained. The explanation usually given is that the change in haemodynamics with the occlusion of a pulmonary artery and the loss of pressure in the occluded vessels causes a retrograde flow of blood in the pulmonary veins and a greater permeability of the walls of the bronchial arteries. However, it fails to explain why in certain instances thromboembolism is not associated with infarction.

It has been estimated that only 10% of all pulmonary thromboembolic episodes result in infarction. Why this is so is not clear. It has been postulated that infarction does not occur in the normal individual because the haemodynamics of the collateral circulation prevent it. Without infarction the lack of blood flow distal to the vascular occlusion cannot be visualized on plain chest X-ray – the radiographic appearance of the chest will be normal.

The healing of an infarct is well documented. If the necrotic infarcted area does not undergo bacterial invasion with resulting abscess formation, the margins of the infarct become revascularized, the occluded vessel is recanalized, the necrotic tissue is slowly absorbed and is eventually replaced by granulation tissue resulting in a linear scar. This can be seen on plain radiographs.

References

1. Allison, P. R., Dunnill, M. S. and Marshall, R. (1960). Pulmonary embolism. *Thorax,* **15,** 273
2. Ashford, T. P. and Freiman, D. G. (1967). The role of the endothelium in the initial phases of thrombosis. *Am. J. Pathol.,* **50,** 257
3. Dalen, J. E., Banas, J. S. Jr, Brooks, H. L., Evans, G. L., Paraskos, J. A. and Dexter, L. (1969). Resolution rate of acute pulmonary embolism in man. *N. Engl. J. Med.,* **280,** 1194
4. Dalen, J. E. and Alpert, J. S. (1975). Natural history of pulmonary embolism. *Prog. Cardiovasc. Dis.,* **17**(4), 259
5. Dalen, J. E., Mathur, V. S. and Evans, H. (1966). Pulmonary angiography in experimental pulmonary embolism. *Am. Heart J.,* **72,** 509
6. Davidson, P. H., Armitage, G. H. and McIlveen, D. J. S. (1956). Chronic cor pulmonale due to silent pulmonary embolism. *Lancet,* **2,** 224
7. deTakats, G. (1950). Anticoagulants in surgery. *J. Am. Med. Assoc.,* **142,** 527
8. Fleishner, F. G. (1967). Recurrent pulmonary embolism and cor pulmonale. *N. Engl. J. Med.,* **276,** 1213
9. Fred, H. L., Axelrad, M. A., Lewis, T. M. and Alexander, J. K. (1966). Rapid resolution of pulmonary thromboemboli in man. An angiographic study. *J. Am. Med. Assoc.,* **196,** 1137
10. Freiman, D. G., Suyemoto, J. and Wessler, S. (1965). Frequency of pulmonary thromboembolism in man. *N. Engl. J. Med.,* **272,** 1278
11. Gibbs, N. M. (1957). Venous thrombosis of the lower limbs with particular reference to bed rest. *Br. J. Surg.,* **45,** 209
12. Heitzman, E. R., Markarian, B., Berger, I. and Dailey, E. (1969). The secondary pulmonary lobule. *Radiology,* **93,** 907
13. Hume, M., Sevitt, S. and Thomas, D. P. (1970). *Venous Thrombosis and Pulmonary Embolism.* (Cambridge: Harvard University Press)
14. Morrell, M. T. and Dunnill, M. S. (1968). The post-mortem incidence of pulmonary embolism in a hospital population. *Br. J. Surg.,* **55,** 347
15. Moser, K. M., Guison, M. and Bartimo, E. E. (1973). Resolution rates of

experimental venous thromboemboli. In Moser, K. M. and Stein, M. (eds.). *Pulmonary Thromboembolism*, p. 104. (Chicago: Year Book Publishers, Inc.)

16. Reichel, J. (1977). Pulmonary embolism. *Symposium on Pulmonary Embolism*, **61**, 309
17. Secker-Walker, R. H., Jackson, J. A. and Goodwin, J. (1970). Resolution of pulmonary embolism. *Br. Med. J.*, **4**, 135
18. Sevitt, S. (1974). The structure and growth of valve-pocket thrombi in femoral veins. *J. Clin. Pathol.*, **27**, 517
19. Sharnoff, J. G. Unpublished data
20. Smith, G. T., Dexter, L. and Demmin, G. J. (1965). Post-mortem quantitative studies in pulmonary embolism. In Sasahara, A. A. and Stein, M. (eds.). *Pulmonary Embolic Disease*. (New York: Grune and Stratton)
21. Spaet, T. H. and Zucker, M. B. (1967). Mechanism of platelet formation and role of adenosine diphosphate. *Am. J. Physiol.*, **206**, 1267
22. Tow, D. E. and Wagner, H. N. Jr. (1967). Recovery of pulmonary arterial blood flow in patients with pulmonary embolism. *N. Engl. J. Med.*, **276**, 1053
23. Wessler, S. (1962). Thrombosis in the presence of vascular stasis. *Am. J. Med.*, **33**, 648
24. Wright, H. P. (1965). The measurement of blood flow. *Ann. R. Coll. Surg. Engl.*, **37**, 292
25. The urokinase pulmonary embolism trial (1973). *Circulation*, **47**, Suppl. II

4

Hypercoagulation and Thrombosis

Hypercoagulation[19], a hitherto little accepted, often questioned condition of the blood, refers to an increase in blood-clotting activities. What triggers this mechanism has never been clearly identified[25]; factors V and VIII, increased levels of fibrinogen, accelerated thromboplastin generation and low levels of *in vivo* heparin production have all been suggested as possible producers of hypercoagulation[6]. A decreased level of antithrombin III[18] has also been implicated as a possible cause. The rationale behind the use of heparin to prevent thrombosis in most instances is the belief that heparin potentiates the neutralising action of antithrombin III on activated factor X (Xa), which is in turn responsible for the prevention of the final generation of thrombin.

More recently, attention has again been directed at the role of platelets[5,20,29,42] in the formation of all thrombi, venous and arterial. The studies of Zahn[49] and Bizzozero[2] in the latter part of the last century demonstrated that platelets were the chief component of the clumped masses in the core of all thrombi. Their adhesiveness appeared to be the main cause of the formation of thrombi in the presence of blood stasis[41]. This has recently prompted most investigators to search for substances which when administered to patients would interfere with platelet function and their adhesiveness. Thus, the use of drugs such as aspirin, dextran[16], hydroxychloroquine, sulfinpyrazone and more recently flurbiprofen[16,21] have been tried all with limited and often contradictory results.

Whatever success has been obtained with these substances indicates that platelets play some role in the formation of intravascular blood clotting. Just what this role is is not entirely clear.

Another platelet phenomenon which prompted the author's most successful programme in prophylaxis of deep vein thrombosis[35] and fatal pulmonary thromboembolism is worthy of inclusion here, although it is not generally accepted and has been described as 'not passing muster'[48]. Yet, an appreciation of this phenomenon has resulted in a rationale for the development of the programme and its safe administration. The initial observation by the author in 1956[29] of escaped bone marrow megakaryocytes entrapped in the pulmonary vessels was followed by a series of further studies[30-33] on animals and humans, which disclosed the manner in which these cells produced a thrombocytosis associated with shortened coagulation times. Following the original observation[30] it could be shown by histochemical means that these entrapped giant cells were truly megakaryocytes found routinely in the capillaries of all lung tissue sections of all mammals, animals and humans in limited numbers[30]. Also, increased numbers of entrapped megakaryocytes could be observed in lung tissue sections of hibernating animals and in inactive or immobilized individuals[34,35]. When the animals or humans were subjected to stress, as in the handling of the animals, or during surgery in humans, this was associated with elevated blood pressure and rapid heart rate. This caused the rapid division of the megakaryocytes in the anastomoses of the lung capillaries into platelets producing a thrombocytosis with simultaneous shortened coagulation times. Using patients under stress from major surgery it could be demonstrated[35] that this period is most critical for thrombocytosis and hypercoagulation. The study also demonstrated that the first period of reactivation of the patient following postoperative immobilization is the second critical period for thrombocytosis and hypercoagulation. From this study it was concluded that though thrombocytosis could not be avoided, an anticoagulant should prevent hypercoagulation[36]. The study also disclosed that there was no significant difference in the level of thrombocytosis and hypercoagulation between those patients who succumbed to thrombosis and embolism and those who did not.

This prompted the conclusion that only small doses of anticoagulant would suffice to avoid thrombosis and possible fatal pulmonary thromboembolism.

Heparin sodium was chosen as the best anticoagulant available for the purpose. These observations prompted the author's (small dose) heparin sodium regime and served as the basic rationale of a successful programme[38–40]. However, a number of other theoretical explanations have been proposed to explain hypercoagulation. The literature on this subject is confusing. This has been due chiefly to the lack of a reliable coagulation test or tests[9,10,15,43,44] to indicate the changes in coagulation factors which could lead to the recognition of a thrombotic state *in vivo*. As a result there was no evidence that such a condition existed or that it could be predicted.

Coagulation factors – II, VII, X, XI and XII – as well as cofactors fibrinogen and the inhibitors are normally present in large amounts. But as only small amounts are activated during thrombus formation *in vivo*, it is therefore unlikely that increased levels would be a predictor of thrombus formation, or that reduced levels of these coagulation factors would be a sensitive indicator of the presence of a thrombus.

It has also been shown that increased levels of factors V, VIII and fibrinogen are present during inflammation. They are acute phase proteins and are probably a non-specific response to extensive thrombosis or other disease. Increased levels of coagulation factors during pregnancy have also been reported and in women taking oral contraceptives containing oestrogen[1,3,24,28].

Further confusion is added by the many clinical and experimental studies on the activation of the coagulation factors which are likely to produce a thrombogenic state *in vivo*. Most studies have been performed on animals or *in vitro* but elucidation of this mechanism is still lacking.

Wessler and Gitel[48] have demonstrated experimentally that there is a marked difference in thrombogenesis between activated and non-activated clotting factors. Others have shown that a number of biological agents can activate coagulation factors and that factor XII may be activated by collagen, endotoxin and a variety of non-tissue surfaces. It has also been shown that factor X may be activated by mucin as in adenocarcinoma or other malignancies[23,26]. It has been suggested that the release of tissue thromboplastin[11] entering the circulation during trauma, surgery and childbirth as well as in myocardial injury may also activate thrombosis. It has further been suggested that an endotoxin may be the underlying cause of thrombosis in disseminated intravascular coagulation, or that leukaemic leukocytes such as the granulocytes exposed to toxin may release a tissue factor to activate thrombosis. This is offered as an explanation for the consumption coagulopathy associated with acute promyelocytic leukaemia[13,14].

Venous thrombosis has been demonstrated experimentally after the infusion of concentrates of factors II, VII, IX and X. This condition has been observed under certain conditions in man, such as in the postoperative patient[8] and in liver disease. However, these patients may have low levels of antithrombin III which may well lower the protective effect of this factor and induce thrombosis.

More recently a radioimmunoassay for measuring thrombin activity has been attempted, and the immunoelectrophoretic mobility of antithrombin III has also been studied. Both methods are an attempt to determine the development of thrombosis but their value has yet to be determined.

Another approach to pinpoint the occurrence of intravascular clotting has been the determination of a decrease in coagulation factors such as II, V, VII, XI and fibrinogen as well as a reduction in platelets. However, these factors will be reduced in the presence of thrombosis, only when the process is very extensive.

Another insensitive attempt has been the measurement of fibrinogen turnover in order to detect arterial or small venous thrombi; this was done using isotope-labelled fibrinogen.

The measurement of fibrinogen degradation products[6,12,15,17,20] has also been thought useful in the determination of venous thrombosis. Elevated levels were found in thrombosis and pulmonary embolism, but were also observed in inflammatory disease, following surgery, trauma or in the presence of malignancy. As a diagnostic test it is therefore of limited value.

There are a number of circulating inhibitory factors[27,28] which are capable of preventing thrombosis, but when present in reduced quantities may or may not induce thrombosis. The most important of these is antithrombin III, which inhibits activated factors X, XI, XII and thrombin. As mentioned above this inhibition is most marked in the presence of heparin[27].

There appears to be some evidence that naturally occurring heparin is present in the circulation in trace amounts, although difficult to detect except on endothelium. When present in decreased amounts it is believed to induce thrombosis.

Another possible explanation for the development of thrombosis is the possibility of reduced fibrinolytic activity. The latter has been reported in patients with recurrent leg vein thrombosis[20].

The role of platelets in the development of hypercoagulability and thrombosis is generally accepted. (Its activity is discussed more fully in Chapter 5.) Platelets aggregate, adhere to surfaces and release agents which activate coagulation factors such as V, VII, IX and X thereby stimulating the formation of thrombin.

There is little evidence that the so-called 'hyperactive' platelets are the cause of thrombosis. The evidence[29] that freshly formed platelets are derived from the pulmonary megakaryocytes mentioned earlier, and the observed association with the sudden development of thrombocytosis accompanied by shortened coagulation times (hypercoagulation) leading to deep vein thrombosis and pulmonary embolism, has led to the development of any number of platelet function tests. They were devised to demonstrate the role of platelets in hypercoagulation. The tests attempt to measure platelet adhesiveness to glass and/or any foreign surface as well as to collagen. All of these tests appear to have little confirmation and are of limited diagnostic or predictive value.

A greater increase in platelet aggregation in patients with type II hyperproteinaemia[5] in the presence of adrenalin, collagen and ADP has been reported. This too has little clinical application, nor does it prove that there is a causal relationship between platelet function as measured *in vitro* and the development of blood hypercoagulability and thrombosis.

Walsh[45] has reported a significant increase in platelet coagulant activity in postoperative patients who develop thrombosis, as detected by [^{125}I]fibrinogen leg scanning. This has also been observed[46] in patients with transient cerebral ischaemia.

The role of platelet survival and turnover has also been investigated in patients with thromboembolic disease. Reduced platelet survival has been observed in arterial disease, arterial thrombosis, prosthetic heart valve replacement, prosthetic artery grafts, arteriovenous shunts, ischaemic heart disease, and venous thrombosis.

Decreased platelet survival is found more often than not in patients with prosthetic heart valves and aortocoronary bypass[42,47], who after surgery develop thromboembolic complications. Zajtchuk et al.[50] noted hypercoagulable blood levels in their patients with diminished blood flow as measured by low levels of antithrombin III, high thrombin, high factor VIII levels or high platelet adhesivity. If this study is confirmed, the measurement of these parameters in vascular surgery may have significant value.

If only out of this confused picture a single simple explanation would evolve that could be readily understood and applied to a uniform means of anticipating the development of deep vein thrombosis and possible embolism, then a generally accepted standard programme of prophylaxis could evolve, capable of considerably reducing morbidity and mortality. At this time the readily understood and easily applied simple, easily controlled and safe (small dose) heparin sodium regime[29] developed by the author appears to offer this possibility.

References

1. Astedt, B., Isaacson, S. and Nilsson, I. M. (1973). Thrombosis and oral contraceptives: possible predisposition. *Br. Med. J.*, **4**, 631
2. Bizzozero, J. (1880). Ueber einem neuen Formbestandtheil des Blutes und dessen Rolle bei der Thrombose und Blutgerinnung. *Virchow's Arch. Pathol. Anat. Physiol. Klin. Med.*, **90**, 261
3. Bonnar, J., McNicol, G. P. and Douglas, A. S. (1969). Fibrinolytic enzyme system and pregnancy. *Br. Med. J.*, **3**, 387
4. Cade, J., Hirsch, J. and Regoszi, E. (1975). Mechanisms for elevated fibrin/ fibrinogen degradation products in acute experimental pulmonary embolism. *Blood*, **45**, 563
5. Carvalho, A. C. A., Colman, R. W. and Lees, R. S. (1974). Platelet function in hyperproteinemia. *N. Engl. J. Med.*, **290**, 434
6. Cooke, E. D., Gordon, Y. B., Bowcock, S. A., Sola, C. M., Pilcher, M. F., Chard, T., Ibborson, R. M. and Ainsworth, M. E. (1975). Serum fibrin(ogen) degradation products in diagnosis of deep vein thrombosis and pulmonary embolism after hip surgery. *Lancet*, **2**, 51
7. Davie, E. W. and Fukikawa, K. (1975). Basic mechanisms in blood coagulation. *Ann. Rev. Biochem.*, **44**, 799
8. Dechavanne, M., Ville, D., Viale, J. J., Kher, A., Faivre, J., Pousset, M. B. and Dejour, H. (1974). Controlled trial of platelet anti-aggregating agents and subcutaneous heparin in preventiom of postoperative deep vein thrombosis in high risk patients. *Haemostasis*, **4**, 94
9. Fletcher, A. P. and Alkjaersig, N. (1972). Blood screening methods for the diagnosis of venous thrombosis. *Millbank Mem. Fund Q.*, **50**, 170
10. Gallus, A. S., Hirsh, J. and Gent, M. (1973). Relevance of preoperative and postoperative blood tests to postoperative leg vein thrombosis. *Lancet*, **2**, 805
11. Garg, S. K. and Niemetz, J. (1973). Tissue factor activity of normal and leukaemic cells. *Blood*, **42**, 729
12. Gordon-Smith, I. C., Hickman, J. A. and LeQuesne, L. P. (1974). Post-operative fibrinolytic activity and deep vein thrombosis. *Br. J. Surg.*, **61**, 213
13. Gouault-Heilmann, M., Chardon, E., Sultan, C. *et al.* (1975). The pro-

45

coagulant factor of leukaemic promyelocytes. Demonstration of immuno-logical cross reactivity with human brain tissue factor. *Br. J. Haematol.*, **30**, 151

14. Gralnick, H. R. and Sultan, C. (1975). Acute promyelocytic leukaemia: haemorrhagic manifestations and morphological criteria. *Br. J. Haematol.*, **29**, 373

15. Gurewich, V., Hume, M. and Patrick, M. (1973). The laboratory diagnosis of venous thromboembolic disease by measurement of fibrinogen/fibrin degradation products and fibrin monomer. *Chest*, **64**, 585

16. Harris, W. H., Salzman, E. W., Athanasoulis, C. A., Waltman, A.C., Baum, S. and DeSanctis, R. W. (1974). Comparison of warfarin, low-mol-ecular weight dextran, aspirin and subcutaneous heparin prevention of ven-ous thromboembolism following total hip replacement. *J. Bone Jt. Surg.*, **56A**, 1552

17. Hedner, U. and Nilsson, I. M. (1971). Clinical experience with determination of fibrinogen degradation products. *Acta Med. Scand.*, **189**, 471

18. Hedner, U. and Nilsson, I. M. (1973). Antithrombin III in a clinical ma-terial. *Thromb. Res.*, **3**, 631

19. Hirsh, J. (1977). Hypercoagulability. *Semin. Hematol.*, **14**, 409

20. Isaacson, S. and Nilsson, I.M. (1972). Defective fibrinolysis in blood and vein walls in recurrent 'idiopathic' vein thrombosis, *Acta Chir. Scand.*, **138**, 313

21. Morris, G. K. and Mitchell, J. R. A. (1977). Preventing venous thrombo-embolism in elderly patients with hip fractures; studies of low-dose heparin, dipyridamole, aspirin and flurbiprofen. *Br. Med. J.*, **1**, 535

22. O'Brien, J. R., Tulovski, V. G., Etherington, M., Madgwick, T., Alkjaersig, N. and Fletcher, A. (1974). Platelet function studies before and after oper-ation and the effect of postoperative thrombosis. *J. Lab. Clin. Med.*, **83**, 342

23. Pineo, G. F., Brain, M. C., Gallus, A. S. *et al.* (1974). Tumors, mucus production and hypercoagulability. *Ann. NY Acad. Sci.*, **230**, 262

24. Poller, L., Thomson, J. M. and Thomas, J. M. (1971). Oestrogen, progester-one, oral contraception and blood clotting. A long term follow up. *Br. Med. J.*, **4**, 648

25. Ratnoff, O. D. (1973). The hypercoagulable state. In Moser, K. M. and Stein, M. (eds.). *Pulmonary Embolism*, p. 3. (Chicago: Year Book Medical Publishers Inc.)

26. Rennie, J. A. N. and Ogston, D. (1975). Fibrinolytic activity in malignant disease. *J. Clin. Pathol.*, **28**, 872

27. Rosenberg, R. D. (1975). Actions and interactions of antithrombin and heparin. *N. Engl. J. Med.*, **292**, 146

28. Sagar, S., Stamatakis, J. D. and Thomas, D. P. (1976). Oral contraceptives, antithrombin III activity and postoperative deep vein thrombosis. *Lancet*, **1**, 509

29. Sharnoff, J. G. (1957). Thrombotic thrombocytopenic purpura. *Am. J. Med.*, **23**, 740

30. Sharnoff, J. G. and Kim, E. S. (1958). Evaluation of pulmonary megakaryo-cytes. *Arch. Pathol.*, **66**, 176

31. Sharnoff, J. G. and Kim, E. S. (1958). Pulmonary megakaryocyte studies in rabbits. *Arch. Pathol.*, **66**, 340
32. Sharnoff, J. G. (1959). Increased pulmonary megakaryocytes – probable role in postoperative thromboembolism. *J. Am. Med. Assoc.*, **169**, 688
33. Sharnoff, J. G. and Scardino, V. (1959). Pulmonary megakaryocytes in human fetuses and premature and full term infants. *Arch. Pathol.*, **69**, 139
34. Sharnoff, J. G. and Scardino, V. (1960). Platelet count differences in blood of rabbit right and left heart ventricles. *Nature (London)*, **187**, 334
35. Sharnoff, J. G., Bagg, J. F., Breen, S. R., Rogliano, A. G., Walsh, A.R. and Scardino, V. (1960). The possible indication of postoperative thromboembolism by platelet counts and blood coagulation studies in patients undergoing extensive surgery. *Surg. Gynecol. Obstet.*, **111**, 469
36. Sharnoff, J. G., Kass, H. H. and Mistica, B. A. (1962). A plan of heparinization of the surgical patient to prevent postoperative thromboembolism. *Surg. Gynecol. Obstet.*, **115**, 75
37. Sharnoff, J. G. (1966). Results in the prophylaxis of postoperative thromboembolism. *Surg. Gynecol. Obstet.*, **123**, 303
38. Sharnoff, J. G. and DeBlasio, G. (1970) Prevention of fatal postoperative thromboembolism by heparin prophylaxis. *Lancet*, **2**, 1006
39. Sharnoff, J. G. (1973). Prevention of thromboembolism. *Bull. NY Acad. Med.*, **49**, 655
40. Sharnoff, J. G., Rosen, R. L., Sadler, A. H. and Ibarra-Isunza, G. C. (1976). Prevention of fatal thromboembolism by heparin prophylaxis after surgery for hip fractures, *J. Bone Jt. Surg.*, **58A**, 913
41. Sherry, S. (1975). Low-dose heparin prophylaxis for postoperative venous thromboembolism. *N. Engl. J. Med.*, **293**, 300
42. Steele, P. P. Weily, H. S. and Genton, E. (1973). Platelet survival and adhesiveness in recurrent venous thrombosis. *N. Engl. J. Med.*, **288**, 1148
43. Tibbutt, D. A., Chesterman, C. N., Allington, M. J., Williams, E. W. and Faulkner, T. (1975). Measurement of fibrinogen–fibrin related antigen in serum as aid to deep vein thrombosis in out-patients. *Br. J. Med.*, **1**, 367
44. Vreeken, J., van der Meer, J., Fedder, G. *et al.* (1974). Chronic fibrinaemia as an indicator of a prethrombotic state. *Neth. J. Med.*, **17**, 121
45. Walsh, P. N. (1975). Role of platelets in pathogenesis of venous thrombosis, prophylactic therapy of deep vein thrombosis and pulmonary embolism. *National Institute of Health DHEW* Publication 76–866, p. 60
46. Walsh, P. N., Paret, F. I. and Corbett, J. J. (1976). Platelet coagulant activities and serum lipids and transient ischemia. *N. Engl. J. Med.*, **295**, 854
47. Weily, H. S., Steele, P. P., Davies, H., Pappas, G. and Genton, E. (1974). Platelets survival in patients with substitute heart valves. *N. Engl. J. Med.*, **290**, 534
48. Wessler, S. and Gitel, S. (1976). Control of heparin therapy. *Hemostas. Thromb.*, **3**, 311
49. Zahn, F. W. (1875). Untersuchungen ueber Thrombose: Bildung der Thromben. *Virchow's Arch. Pathol. Anat. Physiol. Klin. Med.*, **62**, 81
50. Zajtchuk, R., Collins, G. I., Holley, P. W., Heydorn, W. H., Schuchman, G. F. and Homaker, W. R. (1977). Coagulation factors influencing thromboses of aorta-coronary bypass grafts. *J. Thorac. Cardiovasc. Surg.*, **73**, 307

5

Pharmacology of Platelets

It is still uncertain just what role platelets play in the development of thrombosis[45] but it is generally agreed that the aggregation of platelets and the release of thrombin is the coagulation pathway to thrombosis[6]. Thrombin also converts fibrinogen to fibrin, an essential element in the fixation of the platelet aggregate into a thrombus. Substances which effectively prevent the formation of the enzyme thrombin are heparin[19] and the coumarins[23]; they are the most useful agents for the prevention of venous thrombosis and pulmonary embolism.

There are a number of *in vivo* agents which cause platelets to change their shape to a more rounded form with pseudopods. These altered forms can cause them to adhere to each other and release their granular contents[40]. It is likely that the platelets have specific receptors for the aggregating agents, the chief *in vivo* being thrombin, collagen, adenosine diphosphate (ADP), serotonin, epinephrine, antigen–antibody complexes, platelet isoantibodies, bacteria and viruses[39].

It may well be that agents which induce the release[42] reaction in platelets activate a phospholipase which catalyses a coagulation system from platelet phospholipids. The cyclo-oxygenase of platelets in turn catalyses the conversion of this arachidonate system to prostaglandin which in turn gives way to thromboxane A_2[33,40]. These are believed to be unstable intermediates of prostaglandin metabolism and are aggregating and release-inducing agents[33,34,40].

It has been shown that adenosine diphosphate (ADP) is one of the substances in platelet granules released when platelets are exposed to agents such as collagen and thrombin. It may well be that ADP is lost from injured cells which in the presence of calcium induces platelet aggregation[40]. Deaggregation, however, follows rapidly unless the aggregates are stabilized by the formation of fibrin. It would appear unlikely that ADP by itself activates phospholipase or causes the release reaction *in vivo*.

The role of serotonin in the formation of thrombi is not clear. However, it has been shown[33] to stimulate other aggregating agents. Platelet aggregates induced by serotonin deaggregate rapidly and do not undergo the release reaction.

Low concentrations of collagen causing platelet aggregation appear to be induced by released ADP, but this may be blocked with aspirin. On the other hand, thrombin aggregation of platelets is not blocked by released ADP. All of the above are based on *in vitro* studies; these phenomena have not been studied in any great detail *in vivo*. It would appear likely that the antigen–antibody complexes act in the same way as collagen. Some viruses are similar to thrombin in their effect on platelet aggregation[26].

It is more likely that platelet aggregation *in vivo* is induced by several aggregating and release-inducing agents acting in combination. Concentrations of ADP and thrombin alone may be weak aggregating agents but together they can cause marked platelet aggregation. Other combinations of aggregating agents with a similar effect may be collagen and thrombin, and also prostaglandin and thrombin.

Most tests of platelet function as performed *in vitro* are of limited value for the determination of susceptibility to thrombosis or the potential use of antiplatelet drugs. Mustard, Rowsell and Murphy[37] are of the opinion that platelet survival and turnover is one of the few tests of platelet function that has demonstrated a good correlation with clinical manifestations of thromboembolic phenomena.

Drugs such as dipyridamole and sulphinpyrazone have been shown to prolong platelet survival. These drugs have not demonstrated any inhibitory effect on platelet aggregation. Aspirin, however, which has an inhibitory effect on platelet aggregation and release in response to collagen, ADP or epinephrine *in vitro* has not been shown to prolong platelet survival in humans[11].

Drugs which inhibit the function of platelets and the formation of thrombin are therefore of potential value in the prevention of thrombosis and pulmonary thromboembolism. The most important of these are heparin, dipyridamole[2,9] and anti-inflammatory agents[11,39] such as aspirin. A number of other agents as yet not fully evaluated have also shown some potential[7,9–11,13,16,17,22].

Heparin[19,44] in large doses has been shown to prevent thrombus formation by interacting with antithrombin III and so inhibiting the effect of thrombin. It appears to have both an anticoagulant and an antiplatelet effect and as a powerful anticoagulant it has a tendency to cause bleeding. In high concentrations heparin prevents the interaction of platelets with collagen. Clinically it has been shown to be highly effective in preventing venous thrombosis and pulmonary embolism. This has been confirmed by a recent international multicentre trial in which a fixed dose regime of (low dose) heparin prevented fatal pulmonary thromboembolism. There is also some evidence that heparin is effective in the prevention of coronary artery thrombosis[44]. However, long-term trials are required to confirm the latter.

Dipyridamole does inhibit platelet aggregation and the platelet-release reaction induced by many aggregating agents. Its mode of action is unclear, however, although it does prevent platelet adhesion to collagen. But prostaglandin E_1 produces the same effect, and at present it is not clear whether dipyridamole has a direct or indirect effect[2,9,18,22,38].

Dipyridamole in animal studies can, it appears, prolong bleeding time. It appears to diminish and lessen thrombus formation at points of vessel injury and to reduce platelet microaggregation. It has also been shown to prevent shortening of platelet survival. Most experimental evidence indicates that this drug is an effective inhibitor of the interaction of platelets on damaged vessel walls.

In humans, dipyridamole has not been found to have any effect on the survival of patients who had myocardial infarctions[22]. Most reports indicate that dipyridamole was ineffective in preventing venous thrombosis in patients undergoing hip surgery[35]. It did not alter the frequency of ischaemic cerebral episodes[2]. It would appear that the effectiveness of dipyridamole has not been proven and that additional well controlled studies are necessary to determine its value in preventing thrombosis. Administered usually as a 400 mg/day dose in most studies, in 25% of patients its side-effects cause nausea, vomiting and headaches[38].

Hydroxychloroquine[10,13], the antimalarial agent, has been shown to have anti-inflammatory properties and is able to inhibit platelet aggregation by ADP or collagen and the release reaction produced by thrombin or collagen. Chrisman et al.[13], reporting on the use of hydroxychloroquine in 600 mg daily doses in orthopaedic surgery reduced the incidence of deep vein thrombosis. However, further evaluation is necessary to establish its efficacy.

Anti-inflammatory drugs such as aspirin, sulphinpyrazone, phenylbutazone and indomethacin inhibit collagen-induced platelet aggregation and the second phase of aggregation produced by ADP or epinephrine in citrated human platelet-rich plasma. These drugs inhibit the cyclo-oxygenase of platelets and block the formation of prostaglandins which induce the formation of thromboxane A_2[40]. These substances can inhibit the changes of platelet shape, aggregation and the release reaction in experimental conditions, and they have been shown to inhibit platelet adhesion to subendothelial structures. In test systems, aspirin has been shown to be ineffective[35], whereas sulphinpyrazone and indomethacin show some inhibition of platelet adherence to these surfaces. It has also been reported that in flowing blood, aspirin has no effect on platelet adherence to the subendothelial layers.

Administered in humans these drugs appear to have a different effect from that in experimental animals. Sulphinpyrazone[3] lengthens platelet survival and aspirin administered at 3 g/day does not. In platelet-rich plasma, aspirin has been shown to inhibit collagen-induced aggregation while sulphinpyrazone[4] has no effect. Aspirin can prolong bleeding time in man while sulphinpyrazone does not. It may well be that the inhibition of the effect of collagen on platelets is responsible for the prolonged bleeding time induced by aspirin.

These drugs are weak inhibitors of thrombin-induced platelet aggregation and the release reaction. Therefore, if thrombin plays a significant role in thrombus formation it is very unlikely that any of these drugs, particulary aspirin, have much effect on the process. It has been shown that moderate doses of aspirin (1 g/day) has no effect on venous thrombus formation whereas higher doses (1.5–3.6 g/day) may prevent thrombosis. How this is effected is not clear, since aspirin does not seem to have an important effect on blood coagulation. This is supported by the observations of Hennekens, Karlson and Rosner[25] who in a retrospective study found little benefit from the use of aspirin in the prevention of coronary deaths. They suggested waiting for the results of the Amis trial of J. L. Marks before a final conclusion be drawn.

McSherry[35] on the other hand claims that aspirin, in addition to its antiplatelet effect, also interferes with the hepatic synthesis of vitamin K clotting proteins and may thus have an anticoagulant effect as well. However, there is much disagreement in the literature as to the prophylactic efficacy of aspirin in the prevention of thromboembolism when used in the recommended doses[8,14,18–21,27,29,30,38,39,41,43,45,47].

Harris[24] found aspirin to be effective in hip surgery in preventing thromboembolism in males but not in females, whereas Stamatakis et al.[45] reported no benefit from aspirin in preventing postoperative deep vein thrombosis in patients undergoing total hip replacement.

A number of additional agents not yet fully evaluated, which affect platelet function, include propranolol, hydrocortisone[39], clofibrate[12], and halofenate[17], penicillin and carbenicillin, cyproheptadine, vitamin E, furosemide and prostaglandins[23].

Propranolol appears to inhibit platelet aggregation to collagen by reducing the increased platelet sensitivity to ADP-induced aggregation. Despite the fact that its action is not clear, it appears to improve exercise tolerance in patients with angina pectoris, whereas aspirin does not.

Hydrocortisone may inhibit platelet aggregation and the release action induced by ADP, epinephrine, collagen, thrombin and endotoxin. The mechanism of its inhibition has not been clarified.

Clofibrate and halofenate, the serum lipid lowering agents, inhibit both collagen-induced and ADP aggregation as well as prolong platelet survival. In man they are believed to lower the incidence of myocardial infarctions but not to decrease mortality in patients with proven myocardial infarction[16]. There is no evidence that they have any effect on venous thrombosis.

Penicillin G and carbenicillin inhibit platelet aggregation and the release reaction caused by many aggregating agents. They reduce platelet adhesion, but in high doses they may cause a tendency towards bleeding. They appear to act by coating the surface of platelets and interfering with their function.

The antihistamine, cyproheptadine, also inhibits platelet aggregation and the release reaction produced by most aggregating reagents. It has been used in preventing platelet aggregation in renal transplants and in vascular shunts.

Vitamin E may inhibit platelet aggregation induced by collagen, ADP or epinephrine. Although its mode of action is not clear, it would appear to affect the secondary manner of platelet aggregation and not the primary mechanism.

Furosemide, the diuretic, inhibits the action of platelets to produce prostaglandin endoperoxides and thromboxane A_2, which may explain its ability to inhibit the release reaction.

Prostaglandins such as E_1, D_2 and I_2 appear to be potent inhibitors of platelet aggregation and the release reaction and they may also change the fatty acid composition of the platelets. Much more investigative work is needed to evaluate their action. It may well be that the prostaglandins formed by the platelets reflect a change in the platelet function. The increased sensitivity to aggregating agents in patients with arterial thrombosis and recurrent venous thrombosis may be as a result of the greater ability of platelets to form prostaglandin endoperoxides.

Combinations of some of the above-mentioned drugs[18] may have greater effect than the drugs administered singly. Thus the combination of such drugs as the oral anticoagulants or heparin with drugs that inhibit platelet function may cause greater anticoagulation.

The combined effect of drugs which inhibit platelet functions have been observed. Dipyridamole and aspirin[18] have been noted to potentiate each other's inhibitory effect on thrombosis in small vessels, although there are contradictory observations of the effect of this drug combination on venous thrombosis. Both drugs have a different action on platelet functions and may account for the possible enhanced effect on coagulation.

White and Heptinstall[49] conclude that we still do not know whether damage to the endothelium is the main or only initiator of thrombus formation or whether the activity of platelets *in vitro* has any relationship to their action *in vivo*. These authors are of the opinion that the platelet release reaction is central to thrombosis and provides the means of platelet aggregation, procoagulant activity and platelet adhesiveness to injured endothelium or exposed subendothelium. Therefore, inhibitors of this release reaction such as aspirin or sulphinpyrazone should have a considerable antithrombotic activity. Results with these drugs are, however, still equivocal[47].

What emerges most clearly from the above research is that heparin remains the one antithrombotic agent against which all others should be measured.

References

1. Abrahamsen, A. F. (1968). Platelet survival studies in man with special reference to thrombosis and arteriosclerosis. *Scand. J. Haematol.*, **3**, Suppl. 1
2. Acheson, J., Danta, G. and Hutchinson, E. C. (1969). Controlled trial of dipyridamole in cerebral vascular disease. *Br. Med. J.*, **1**, 614
3. Ali, M. and McDonald, J. W. D. (1977). Effects of sulfinpyrazone on platelet prostaglandin synthesis and platelet release of serotonin. *J. Lab. Clin. Med.*, **89**, 868
4. Anturane Reinfarction Trial Research Group (1978). Sulfinpyrazone in the prevention of cardiac death after myocardial infarction. *N. Engl. J. Med.*, **298**, 289
5. Baumgartner, H. R. (1973). Adhaesion der plaettchen on des subendotheliale gewehe. *Bull. Schweiz. Akad. Med. Wiss.*, **29**, 177
6. Biggs, R., Denson, K. W. E., Riesenberg, D. *et al.* (1968). The coagulant activity of platelets. *Br. J. Haematol.*, **15**, 283
7. Blakeley, J. A. and Pogoviller, G. (1977). A prospective trial of sulfinpyrazone after peripheral vascular surgery. *Thromb. Haemostas.*, **38**, 238
8. Boston Collaborative Drug Surveillance Group (1974). Regular aspirin intake and acute myocardial infarction. *Br. Med. J.*, **1**, 440
9. Browse, N. L. and Hall, J. H. (1969). Effect of dipyridamole on the incidence of clinically detectable deep vein thrombosis. *Lancet*, **2**, 718
10. Carter, A. E. and Eban, R. (1974). Prevention of postoperative deep venous thrombosis in legs by orally administered hydroxychloroquine sulphate. *Br. Med. J.*, **3**, 94
11. Cazenave, J. P., Packham, M. A., Guccione, M. A. and Mustard, J. F. (1974). Inhibition of platelet adherence to a collagen-coated surface by non-steroidal anti-inflammatory drugs pyrimido-pyrimidine and tricyclic compounds and lidocaine. *J. Lab. Clin. Med.*, **83**, 797
12. Chakrabarti, R., Fearnley, G. R. and Evans, J. F. (1968). Effects of clofibrate on fibrinolysis, platelet stickiness plasma-fibrinogen and serum cholesterol. *Lancet*, **2**, 1007
13. Chrisman, O. D., Snook, G. A., Wilson, T. C. and Short, J. Y. (1976).

Prevention of venous thromboembolism by administration of hydroxychloroquine. *J. Bone Jt. Surg.*, **58A**, 918

14. Clagett, G. P., Schneider, P., Rosoff, C. B. and Salzman, E. (1975). The influence of aspirin on postoperative platelet kinetics and venous thrombosis. *Surgery*, **77**, 61

15. Clagett, G. P. and Collins, J. C. (1978). Platelets, thromboembolism and the clinical utility of anti-platelet drugs. *Surg. Gynecol. Obstet.*, **147**, 257

16. Coronary Drug Project Research Group (1975). Clofibrate and niacin in coronary heart disease. *J. Am. Med. Assoc.*, **231**, 360

17. Colman, R. W. Bennett, J. S., Sheridan, J. F., Cooper, R. A., and Shattil, S. J. (1976). Halofenate. A potent inhibitor of normal and hypersensitive platelets. *J. Lab. Clin. Med.*, **88**, 282

18. Dale, J., Myhre, E. and Rootwelt, K. (1975). Effects of dipyridamole and acetylsalicylic acid on platelet functions in patients with aortic ball-valve prosthesis. *Am. Heart J.*, **89**, 613

19. Dechavanne, M., Ville, D., Viale, J. J., Kher, A., Faivre, J., Pousset, M. B. and Dejour, H. (1975). Controlled trial of platelet anti-aggregating agents and subcutaneous heparin in prevention of postoperative deep vein thrombosis in high risk patients. *Haemostasis*, **4**, 94

20. Elwood, P. C., Cochrane, A. L., Burr, M. L., Sweetnam, P. M., Williams, G., Welsby, E., Hughes, S. J. and Renton, R. (1974). A randomized controlled trial of acetylsalicylic acid in the secondary prevention of mortality from myocardial infarction. *Br. Med. J.*, **1**, 436

21. Frishman, W. H., Christodoulou, J., Weksler, B., Smithen, C., Killip, T., and Scheidt, S. (1976). Aspirin therapy in angina pectoris: effects on platelet aggregation, exercise tolerance and electrocardiographic manifestations of ischemia. *Am. Heart J.*, **92**, 3

22. Gent, A. E., Brook, C. G., Foley, T. H. and Miller, T. N. (1968). Dipyridamole: a controlled trial of its effect in acute myocardial infarction. *Br. Med. J.*, **4**, 366

23. Genton, E., Gent, M., Hirsh, J. and Harker, L. (1975). Platelet inhibiting drugs in the prevention of clinical thrombotic disease. *N. Engl. J. Med.*, **293**, 1296

24. Harris, W. H. (1977). Aspirin prophylaxis against thromboembolic disease. *Thromb. Haemostas.*, **38**, 236

25. Hennekens, C. H., Karlson, L. K. and Rosner, B. (1978). A case control study of regular aspirin use and coronary deaths. *Circulation*, **58**, 35

26. Hirsh, J., Street, D., Cade, J. F. and Amy, H. (1973). Relation between bleeding time and platelet connective tissue reaction after aspirin. *Blood*, **41**, 369

27. Hume, M., Bierbaum, B., Kuriakose, T. X. and Suprenant, J. (1977). Prevention of postoperative thrombosis by aspirin. *Am. J. Surg.*, **133**, 420

28. Jennings, J. J., Harris, W. H. and Sormiento, A. (1976). A clinical evaluation of aspirin prophylaxis of thromboembolic disease after total hip arthroplasty. *J. Bone Jt. Surg.*, **58A**, 926

29. Jobin, F. (1978). Acetylsalicylic acid, hemostasis and human thromboembolism. *Semin. Thromb. Hemostas.*, **4**, 3

30. Justice, C., Papavangelou, E. and Edwards, W. S. (1974). Prevention of

thrombosis with agents which reduce platelet adhesiveness. *Ann. Surg.*, **40**, 186

31. Kaegi, A., Pineo, G. F., Shimizu, A., Trivedi, H., Hirsh, J., and Gent, M. (1974). Arteriovenous shunt thrombosis, prevention by sulfinpyrazone. *N. Engl. J. Med.*, **290**, 304

32. Karapatkin, S., Khan, O. and Freedman, M. (1978). Heterogenicity of platelet function – correlation with platelet volume. *Am. J. Med.*, **64**, 542

33. Kinlough-Rathbone, R. L., Packham, M. A. and Mustard, J. F. (1976). Synergism between platelet aggregating agents: the role of prostaglandin endoperoxides and thromboxane A_2. *Circulation*, **54**, Suppl. 2, 196

34. Lagarde, M. and Dechavanne, M. (1977). Increase of platelet prostaglandin cyclic endoperoxides in thrombosis. *Lancet*, **2**, 88

35. McSherry, J. A. (1978). Deep-vein thrombosis after hip replacement. *Br. Med. J.*, **1**, 1551

36. Moncada, S., Higgs, E. A. and Vane, J. R. (1977). Human arterial and venous tissues generate prostacyclin (prostaglandin X), a potent inhibitor of platelet aggregation. *Lancet*, **1**, 18

37. Mustard, J. F., Rowsell, H. C. and Murphy, E. A. (1966). Platelet economy (platelet survival and turnover). *Br. J. Haematol.*, **12**, 1

38. Oblath, R. W., Buckley, F. O. Jr., Green, R. M., Schwartz, S. I. and DeWeese, J. A. (1978). Prevention of platelet aggregation and adherence to prosthetic vascular grafts by aspirin and dipyridamole. *Surgery*, **84**, 37

39. O'Brien, J. R., Finch, W. and Clark, E. (1970). A comparison of an effect of different anti-inflammatory drugs on human platelets. *J. Clin. Pathol.*, **23**, 522

40. Packham, M. A. and Mustard, J. F. (1977). Clinical pharmacology of platelets. *Blood*, **50**, 555

41. Report of the Steering Committee of a Trial Sponsored by the Medical Research Council (1972). Effect of aspirin on postoperative venous thrombosis. *Lancet*, **2**, 441

42. Salzman, E. W., Lindon, J. and Brier, G. L. *et al.* (1977). Surface induced platelet adhesion, aggregation and release. *Ann. NY Acad. Sci.*, **283**, 114

43. Schondorf, T. H. (1975). Wirkung von acetylsalicyl-lysin auf die thrombocyten Function. *Klin. Wochenschr.*, **53**, 1125

44. Sharnoff, J. G. and DeBlasio, G. (1970). Some implications in the successful prophylaxis of sudden cardio-pulmonary arrest by thrombosis and embolism. *Am. Heart J.*, **80**, 848

45. Stamatakis, J. D., Kakkar, V. V., Lawrence, D., Bentley, P. G., Nairn, D. and Ward, V. (1978). Failure of aspirin to prevent post-operative deep vein thrombosis in patients undergoing total hip replacement. *Br. Med. J.*, **1**, 1031

46. Steele, P. P., Weily, H. S. and Genton, E. (1973). Platelet survival and adhesiveness in recurrent venous thrombosis. *N. Engl. J. Med.*, **288**, 1148

47. Verstrate, M. (1976). Are agents affecting platelet functions clinically useful? *Am. J. Med.*, **61**, 897

48. Weiss, H. J. (1978). Properties of platelets. *N. Engl. J. Med.*, **298**, 1344

49. White, A. M. and Heptinstall, S. (1978). Contribution of platelets to thrombus formation. *Br. Med. Bull.*, **34**, 123

6

Pharmacology of Heparin

Heparin was first discovered by McLean[27] in 1916, who called it cephalin, and it was later named heparin by Howell and Holt[17] in 1918. It has been the object of considerable study as the first available anticoagulant in medicine. It has remarkable multiple pharmacological properties, and as a compatible physiological substance does not cause respiratory complications or cardiovascular shock. It has proved to be a most valuable agent in the treatment and prevention of thrombosis and thromboembolism. It has many other properties which make it extremely valuable as both a direct and indirect anticoagulant agent apart from other clinical uses. For a more complete discussion, the reader is referred to the excellent reviews of L. B. Jaques[20-22].

It was Fischer[15] who demonstrated that heparin binds with proteins thereby modifying their biological activity. Jorpes[24] discovered that heparin was a sulphated polysaccharide; it is also a strongly acid substance. Among its other properties are its ability to: (1) release or activate enzymes such as lipoprotein enzymes; (2) inhibit hormones such as cortisone and aldosterone; (3) detoxify toxic substances; (4) bind histamine in body cells; and (5) give metachromatic reaction, i.e. a specific colour reaction with certain dyes.

Heparin is produced by the mast cells[34] and is demonstrable in extremely small quantities in circulating blood. It was Howell who first purified it from dog liver and thus named it heparin. It was later shown to be obtainable from many mammalian species including the hog, sheep, rats and cattle[5,21,22]. At first the greatest activity was found to be present in the dog, until it was also discovered to have even greater activity in the whale. The substance derived from these animals demonstrated differences in solubility. The molecular weight of heparin has been reported as ranging from 8000 to 19 700 with a mean of 11 900, but heparin forms complexes with many substances such as proteins, by ionic bonds to form salts and non-ionic forces such as the hydrogen bond.

There appears to be a close association between histamine and heparin. In shock situations both are released, and histamine seems to be capable of neutralizing the anticoagulant action of heparin.

The metachromatic property of heparin depends on its ability to combine with dyes that have free amino groups[20]. This reaction is most marked with Toluidine Blue which changes from blue to red. Other dyes giving a metachromatic reaction are: Azure A, Bismarck Brown, Brilliant Cresyl Blue, Neutral Red and Basic Fuchsin. The colour change can be suppressed by heat and alcohol and produced in dilute aqueous solutions, paper chromatography and in tissue sections. The staining is observed in connective tissue, cartilage and the mast cells.

Heparin combines with plasma proteins such as fibrinogen, globulins and albumin, a combination dependent on the concentration of heparin, salts present and pH. Heparin appears to be specific for cryofibrinogen and Waldenstrom's macroglobulin, and it appears to precipitate the beta-lipoprotein fraction[9]. This has been used as a method for the quantitative determination of this fraction.

There are a number of bases which block some of the actions of heparin, in particular anticoagulant, antilipaemic and metachromatic actions, among them. Toluidine Blue, the tetracyclines, stilbadamine and protamine[20]. As there are anti-heparin factors present in the tissues exact quantities of the blockers are necessary to neutralize the activity of heparin.

A number of enzymes are acted upon by heparin, which also has a proteolytic as well as some fibrinolytic activity; small amounts of heparin may activate proteolysis in human serum.

Heparin inhibits fibrinolytic factors directly but not plasmin. It is believed that the effectiveness of heparin on thrombosis is due to the activation of the precursor of fibrinolysin with heparin. It also has no effect on serum or plasma amylase activities. The inhibition of the fibrinolytic effect in plasma by heparin is associated with beta-lipoproteins and may be related to the clearing factor.

The most important relationship of heparin to enzymes is with the lipoprotein lipase, where the action of heparin in the removal of triglycerides from the bloodstream can have a retarding effect on the development of arteriosclerosis[2,6,11,25], although this process still remains an enigma.

Heparin causes some spontaneous haemolysis. It may reverse both the LE reaction in systemic lupus erythematosus and the positive direct and indirect Coombs test. Its success has been reported in the treatment of paroxysmal nocturnal haemoglobinuria[11]. Heparin has also been discovered to interfere with the action of complement.

Heparin has an effect on plant viruses and on the growth of cells in tissue culture, precipitating the mosaic virus of tobacco[20] and retarding cell division in tissue culture.

Heparin may also have an effect on platelets and white blood cells. Heparin appears to cause a thrombocytopenia, but this may be due to a clumping of platelets; it may also produce a leukocytosis[21,31].

Heparin has marked renal effects[13,26,29] causing a moderate and constant diuresis and inhibiting the antidiuretic effect of pitressin. The binding power of intravenous heparin causes a marked increase in potassium excretion, and in patients with oedema, heparin can cause a marked increase in the excretion of sodium chloride and water. Although an antihypertensive agent, it has a different mode of action from other antihypertensives; given subcutaneously it produces a small but lasting decrease in blood pressure.

Heparin has shown to have an inhibitory effect on anaphylactic and sensitivity phenomena. This has been observed in skin allergies, severe asthma and bronchopulmonary disease, as well as in inflammatory disease. The heparin inhibition of allergic reactions may well account for the relatively few instances of sensitization using this therapy. Heparin appears to suppress the appearance of mononuclear cells in inflammatory infiltrations.

The main activity of heparin is anticoagulation[1,3,4,7,10,14,16,19,31]. (This is discussed at greater length in Chapters 9, 10 and 11 on the prevention and therapy of thrombosis.) As this is its most important function it is essential to determine what happens to heparin in the body[13]. Apart from its pharmacological activities, its absorption, distribution, transformation and elimination from the body must be understood before a reasonable schedule of administration is undertaken.

Since an accurate direct chemical assay of heparin in blood is not available, its pharmacokinetics must be studied with methods that measure its action in the blood[13]. The correct method is to measure blood clotting time. There is no evidence that heparin is excreted unchanged in the urine both because it is unlikely that its large molecular size and electronegative charge would permit this, and from the fact that it is bound to plasma protein. Heparin has a half-life of 1½ hours in man[29], but in patients with renal disease, the half-life is prolonged, indicating that in some way the kidneys play a role in its elimination. In normal individuals, however, the tests applied to blood to determine the half-life of heparin action using the activated thromboplastin time (APTT), the partial thromboplastin time (PTT) and Lee–White coagulation time were all in agreement that the half-life was 1½ hours. It is likely that the half-life of heparin may be the most important pharmacokinetic parameter by which heparin therapy can be measured clinically. The clotting time test (which is the simplest, most reproducible, reliable and readily performed at the bedside) is the most desirable[10,14,29]. Of all the whole blood clotting time tests available for this purpose, the Dale and Laidlaw coagulometer, as modified by the author, meets all the above requirements[21].

Despite the reliability of whole blood clotting time tests it is impossible to predict the reaction in any single individual receiving heparin subcutaneously. This has been demonstrated by bioassay[14] and by the pharmacokinetic parameters mentioned above, and in spite of the determination of a baseline obtained before the institution of heparin therapy. There is good evidence that increased doses of heparin are reflected by more prolonged clotting times in most patients receiving heparin therapy. It can be concluded that frequent determinations of the whole blood clotting time tests is essential for determining the heparin needs of any patient receiving heparin so that accurate anticoagulation therapy can be maintained. The reason for the disappearance of heparin from the blood is still not clear[13], as it is not known whether heparin is metabolized or biotransformed. Its rate of disappearance appears to be the same for all doses. This would suggest that the available heparinase enzyme known to be present in blood is insufficient to degrade heparin, and that renal excretion as measured in urine is also insufficient to account for its disappearance. It has been suggested that the heparin plasma half-life as short as 1½ hours may be explained by the transfer of heparin to some extravascular compartment such as the reticuloendothelial system. It has been demonstrated that the reticuloendothelial and connective tissue cells have the ability to participate in the uptake, storage and release of heparin, and this endothelium uptake may be a means of preventing the attachment of platelets to form thrombi. It has also been suggested that heparin may be excreted by the kidneys as uroheparin[26]. It appears that the relatively short half-life is the result of the combined effect of all the methods of elimination mentioned above.

References

1. Abbott, W. M., Warnock, D. F. and Austen, W. G. (1977). The relationship of heparin source to the incidence of delayed hemorrhage. *J. Surg. Res.*, **22**, 593
2. Agostini, B. (1974). The effect of post-heparin lipolytic activity on plasma lipoproteins – a study by electron microscopy. *Histochemistry*, **40**, 215
3. Aiach, M., Flessinger, J. N. and Chousterman, M. (1977). L'heparine. *Rev. Practicien*, **27**, 3953
4. Anderson, L. O., Barrowsliffe, T. W., Holmes, E., Johnson, E. A., and Sims, G. E. C. (1976). Anticoagulant properties of heparin fractionated by affinity chromatography on matrix-bound antithrombin III and by gel filtration. *Thromb. Res.*, **9**, 575
5. Bangham, D. R. and Woodward, P. M. (1970). A collaborative study of heparins from different sources. *Bull. WHO*, **42**, 129
6. Bianchini, P., Isima, B., Rimini, V. and Mocchi, M. (1976). Heparin or heparins? *European Symposium on Advances in Coagulation, Fibrinolysis, Platelet Aggregation and Atherosclerosis*, Palermo, 6–9 Oct., Communication 9
7. Coon, W. H. (1978). Heparin: a drug of varying composition and effectiveness. *Clin. Pharm. Ther.*, **23**, 139
8. Craaford, C. (1937). Preliminary report on post-operative treatment with heparin as a preventative of thrombosis. *Acta Chir. Scand.*, **79**, 407
9. Dahlback, O., Hansson, R., Tibbling, G. and Tryding, N. (1968). The effect of heparin on diamine oxidase and lipoprotein lipase in human lymph and blood plasma. *Scand. J. Clin. Lab. Invest.*, **21**, 17
10. deTakats, G. (1950). Anticoagulants in surgery. *J. Am. Med. Assoc.*, **142**, 527
11. Engelberg, H. (1975). The clinical use of heparin. *Curr. Ther. Res.*, **18**, 34
12. Erdi, A., Kakkar, V. V., Thomas, D. P., Lane, D. A. and Dormandy, J. A. (1976). Effect of low-dose subcutaneous heparin on whole blood viscosity. *Lancet*, **2**, 342
13. Estes, J. W. (1975). The fate of heparin in the body. *Curr. Ther. Res.*, **18**, 45
14. Estes, J. W. (1970). Kinetics of the anticoagulant effect of heparin. *J. Am. Med. Assoc.*, **212**, 1492

15. Fischer, A. (1935). Die bindung von heparin on eiweiss. *Biochem. Z.*, **278**, 133

16. Gallus, A. S., Hirsh, J., O'Brien, S. E., McBride, J. A., Tuttle, R. J. and Gent, M. (1976). Prevention of venous thrombosis with small subcutaneous doses of heparin. *J. Am. Med. Assoc.*, **235**, 1980

17. Howell, W. H. and Holt, E. (1918). Two new factors in blood coagulation – heparin and proantithrombin. *Am. J. Physiol.*, **47**, 328

18. Hiebert, L. M. and Jaques, L. B. (1976). The observation of heparin on endothelium after injection. *Thromb. Res.*, **8**, 195

19. Hirsh, J., VanAken, W. G., Gallus, A. G., Dollery, C. T., Cade, J. F. and Yung, W. L. (1976). Heparin kinetics in venous thrombosis and pulmonary embolism. *Circulation*, **53**, 691

20. Jaques, L. B. and Mahadoo, J. (1978). Pharmacodynamics and clinical effectiveness of heparin. *Semin. Thromb. Hemostas.*, **4**, 298

21. Jaques, L. B. and McDuffie, N. M. (1978). The chemical and anti-coagulant nature of heparin. *Semin. Thromb. Hemostas.*, **4**, 277

22. Jaques, L. B. (1940). The heparins of various mammalian species and their relative anticoagulant potency. *Science*, **92**, 488

23. Johnson, E. A., Kirkwood, T. B. C., Stirling, Y., Perez-Reguejo, J. L., Ingram, G. I. C., Bangham, D. R. and Brozovic, M. (1976). Four heparin preparations: anti-Xa potentiating effect of heparin after subcutaneous injection. *Thromb. Hemostas.*, **35**, 586

24. Jorpes, J. E. (1959). Heparin A mucopolysaccharide and an active antithrombotic drug. *Circulation*, **19**, 87

25. Krauss, R. M., Levy, R. I. and Fredrickson, D. S. (1974). Selective activity of two lipase activities in post-heparin plasma from normal subjects and patients with hyperlipoprotein. *J. Clin. Invest.*, **54**, 1107

26. McAllister, B. M. and Emis, D. J. (1966). Heparin metabolism: isolation and characterization of uroheparin. *Nature (London)*, **212**, 293

27. McLean, J. (1916). The thromboplastic action of cephalin. *Am. J. Physiol.*, **41**, 250

28. Olsson, P., Lagergren, H. and Ek, S. (1963). The elimination from plasma of intravenous heparin, an experimental study on dogs and humans. *Acta Med. Scand.*, **173**, 619

29. Perry, P. J., Herron, G. R. and King, J. C. (1974). Heparin half-life in normal and impaired renal function. *Clin. Pharmacol. Ther.*, **16**, 514

30. Rosenberg, R. D. (1977). Chemistry of the hemostatic mechanism and its relationship to the action of heparin. *Fed. Proc.*, **36**, 10

31. Sharnoff, J. G., Rosen, R. L., Sadler, A. H. and Ibarra-Izunza, G. C. (1976). Prevention of fatal pulmonary thromboembolism by heparin prophylaxis after surgery for hip fractures. *J. Bone Jt. Surg.*, **58A**, 913

32. Silverglade, A. (1975). Biological equivalence of beef lung and hog mucosal heparins. *Curr. Ther. Res.*, **18**, 91

33. Wahl, T. O., Lipshitz, D. A. and Stechschulte, D. J. (1978). Thrombocytopenia associated with antiheparin antibody. *J. Am. Med. Assoc.*, **240**, 2566

34. Yurt, R. W., Leid, R. W., Austin, K. F. and Silbert, J. E. (1977). Native heparin from rat peritoneal mast cells. *J. Biol. Chem.*, **252**, 518

7

Clinical Uses of Heparin

The biochemical properties of heparin have led to a variety of clinical uses. Depending on its concentration, heparin as a highly acid substance binds with one or more proteins thereby altering their action. As a natural body substance, heparin appears to play an important role in the physiological processes of the body.

When first discovered by McLean[19] in 1916 and named cephalin, it was found to have an anticoagulant action which has proved to be its most important clinical value. It is active as an anticoagulant both *in vitro* and *in vivo*. Its activity *in vitro* has led to its successful use in preventing blood from clotting in test tubes, in cardiac surgery where heart–lung machines are necessary[4,6,7] and in haemodialysis of uraemic patients[9].

The most important use of heparin *in vivo* is in the prevention and the treatment of thrombosis. (This is discussed more fully in Chapters 8, 10, 12 and 13.) In the past it has been used chiefly via the intravenous route by intermittent injections or by continuous infusions where it can cause severe and sometimes fatal haemorrhages. The objective with the intravenous method of therapy is to attain clotting times of two to three times the normal control. The subcutaneous administration of heparin, which is currently the generally advocated method of prevention, has the objective of maintaining normocoagulation as indicated by normal controls in the prevention or the further propagation of already existing thrombi. The subcutaneous heparin method is receiving greater acceptance, particularly as the effectiveness of oral anticoagulants has been found to be disappointing.

Although oral anticoagulants are still being used extensively in the prevention of thromboses in the heart and leg veins in patients with acute myocardial infarctions, more and more heparin is administered in small doses subcutaneously for the same purpose. Heparin administered intravenously has an immediate anticoagulant effect whereas subcutaneous heparin reaches a peak anticoagulant effect after 2–3 hours. Oral anticoagulants on the other hand take several days before the full anticoagulant effect is detectable by laboratory control. It is not generally appreciated, however, that a prolonged prothrombin time is not synonymous with anticoagulation. Heparin is therefore advocated in preventing thrombus propagation and in the treatment of both venous and arterial thrombi[1] at any site such as in cerebral[2] and extremity thrombosis. Besides preventing the propagation of coronary artery thrombi and endocardial mural thrombi in acute myocardial infarction, heparin also prevents the development of deep leg vein thrombosis and embolism in those patients[10,23].

Other possible advantages of heparin prophylaxis in patients with acute myocardial infarction is the lipid-clearing action[13] in blood which is believed to improve the transport of oxygen from the blood to the tissues; this may also help limit the size of the myocardial necrosis. The lipaemic clearing action of heparin may also decrease the rate of development of arteriosclerosis, especially coronary arteriosclerosis. Also, in the case of impending coronary artery occlusion with angina pectoris as the presenting symptom, the prompt administration of small doses of heparin has been reported to halt the angina[3]. It is believed likely that the lipid-clearing action of heparin plays a significant role here, as does the decreased platelet adhesiveness. Indeed, it is rather surprising that with the great frequency of this problem, heparin in small doses is not used more often prophylactically.

Another complication of acute myocardial infarction which can be prevented with the use of heparin is the impaired renal function due to tubular necrosis and possible uraemia. Heparin has also been recommended in chronic renal disease[9]. Pulmonary oedema, a further complication of acute myocardial infarction, also appears to be inhibited with heparin prophylaxis.

In general, there has been a great increase in the use of heparin in other diseases and many claims of its beneficial effect have appeared in the literature. Other diseases besides thromboembolism in which heparin therapy may be used successfully include fat embolism, burns[20-22], hypertension, sepsis, drug toxicity, pancreatitis, autoimmune disease, haemolytic anaemias, cancer, diabetes, and glomerulonephritis[14]. It is believed that cerebral thromboembolism or transient ischaemic episodes can be shortened and result in lesser residual effect by preventing further propagation of the thrombus or embolus[2]. There also appears to be good evidence that severe burns heal faster when heparin sodium is applied topically[20,21]. Heparin prophylaxis has been reported to be particularly beneficial in Gram-negative sepsis where disseminated intravascular coagulation is common[14]. The association of cancer of the pancreas and phlebothrombosis is well known, but there is additional clinical and post-mortem evidence that cancer in general is often complicated by deep vein thrombosis and pulmonary embolism. As for acute pancreatitis, glomerulonephritis, autoimmune disease[9] and drug toxicity, there appears to be some evidence that microthrombi may be present with some frequency; these, too, may benefit from heparin therapy[14]. There is good evidence that acute ulcers of the bowel such as the so-called 'stress ulcers', a frequent serious postoperative complication, are caused by small vessel thrombosis and are generally prevented by heparin prophylaxis. It can be stated that, in general, heparin prophylaxis may be most beneficial for all hospitalized, chiefly immobilized patients for whatever illness they may require hospitalization.

With the advent of open heart surgery, such as prosthetic valve and other vascular surgery, the use of heparin prophylaxis by infusion or intermittent administration has become mandatory[1,4,6,7,15,16]. This is especially true when blood comes in contact with artificial surfaces – a foreign surface which does not create the possibility of thrombosis has yet to be discovered. The type of thrombi formed in these devices either in the body or in extracorporeal machines may be red or white thrombi according to whether or not they contain red cells. The red thrombi usually form in slower blood flow such as in veins and the white in rapid blood flow as in arteries. The thrombi may be of microscopic size or larger and are composed of platelet aggregates and fibrin. The problem of foreign surfaces is particularly noticeable with heart–lung machines where the rapid flow of blood damages the platelets causing their aggregation and thrombus formation. The platelet aggregates produce microemboli which cause small infarcts in various organs, especially the brain and lungs. This can explain the morbidity noted following extracorporeal blood circulation. The formation of these platelet aggregates may account for the thrombocytopenia which is observed to last several days after cardiopulmonary bypass. Heparin administered either intravascularly, by infusion, or subcutaneously during the operative procedure is capable of preventing thrombus formation; the dosage usually has to be large and is determined from control times. The same technique is adopted for bypass vascular surgery in order to prevent thrombosis distal to the site of surgery. At the same time the heparinization can prevent deep vein thrombosis and the possibility of pulmonary thromboembolism.

Heparin is also very useful in haemodialysis. As with extracorporeal circulation, if haemodialysis is to be effective there must be a free flow of blood over the dialysing membrane and through the arterial and venous blood tubing connecting the patient to the machine. Again, these foreign surfaces may cause the blood to clot, giving rise to complications. Heparin is therefore used to prevent this tendency during the treatment, and it may be administered systemically by continuous infusions, intermittent injections or regionally[5,11,12]. The dose to be given is generally determined by the patient's body weight and the monitoring control values. When administered as a continuous infusion 1000–2000 USP units/h are given continuously during dialysis with monitoring determining any necessary change in dosage.

When heparin is administered by the intermittent method it is generally injected at regular intervals intravenously or subcutaneously depending on coagulation monitoring values. Maintaining at normal coagulation levels or better may be all that is required.

In regional heparinization, heparin is infused continuously into the arterial blood tubing line that carries blood from the patient to the dialysing membrane. In smaller doses it may not be necessary to infuse protamine sulphate into the venous return line to the patient as the blood may be at normocoagulable levels, thus requiring no neutralization of the heparin. Oral anticoagulants should not be used. Heparin is the drug of choice in the prevention of clotting in the dialyser membrane and the tubing.

Heparin has also been found beneficial in preventing thrombosis in intravenous and intra-arterial catheterization. Here again the artificial surfaces employed in the administration of drugs or electrolyte fluids may give rise to thrombosis and thrombophlebitis. The addition of 1000 units of heparin to the electrolyte fluids has prevented these complications and maintained the viability of the catheters.

Systemic heparinization has also been found beneficial in transfemoral percutaneous arteriography, coronary arteriography and catheterization in the prevention of myocardial infarctions.

Heparin has also been used successfully in the treatment of venous thrombosis and embolism in pregnancy[8,13,18]. Oral anticoagulants should not be used in this condition since coumadin or warfarin can cross the placental barrier and produce fetal malformations. Heparin on the other hand has a large molecule which does not cross the placenta and affect the fetus. Heparin has also been recommended in the dissolution of gallstones[17,24] and has been advocated in the treatment of inflammatory disease, although the evidence to date for the latter conditions appears questionable.

References

1. Antonovic, R., Rosch, J. and Dotter, C. T. (1976). The value of systemic arterial heparinization in transfemoral antiography: a prospective study. *Am. J. Roentgen.*, **127**, 223
2. Baker, R. N., Broward, J. A., Fang, H. C., Fisher, C. M., Groch, S. N., Heyman, A., Karp, H. R., McDevitt, E., Scheinberg, P., Schwartz, W. and Toole, J. F. (1962). Anticoagulant therapy in cerebral infarction. *Neurology*, **12**, 823
3. Bottiger, L.E., Carlson, L. A., Engstedt, L. and Oro, L. (1967). Long term heparin treatment in ischemic heart disease. *Acta Med. Scand.*, **182**, 245
4. Brenner, W. I., Engelman, R. M., Williams, C. D., Boyd, A. D. and Reed, G. E. (1974). Non-thrombogenic aortic and vena caval bypass using heparin-coated tubes. *Rev. Surg.*, **31**, 132
5. Brown, G. (1970). Infusion thrombophlebitis. *Br. J. Clin. Pract.*, **24**, 197
6. Bull, B. S., Korpman, R. A., Huse, W. M. and Briggs, B. D. (1975). Heparin therapy during extracorporeal circulation. I. *J. Thorac. Cardiovasc. Surg.*, **69**, 674
7. Bull, B. S., Huse, W. M., Brauer, E. S. and Korpman, R. A. (1975). Heparin therapy during extracorporeal circulation. II. *J. Thorac. Cardiovasc. Surg.*, **69**, 685
8. Buyse, F. G.C., Wormgoor, B. H., Bernard, J. T. L. and Koudstraal, J. (1974). Anticoagulant therapy with repeated placental infarction. *Obstet. Gynecol.*, **43**, 844
9. Cameron, J. S., Gill, B., Turner, D. R., Chantler, C., Ogg, C. S., Vasnides, G. and Williams, D. G. (1975). Combined immuno-suppression and anticoagulation in rapidly progressive glomerulonephritis. *Lancet*, **2**, 923
10. Chalmers, T.C., Matta, R. J., Smith, Jr., H. and Kunzler, M. A. (1977). *N. Engl. J. Med.*, **297**, 1091
11. Collin, J., Collin, C., Constable, F. L. and Johnston, I. D. A. (1975). Infusion thrombophlebitis and infection with various cannulas. *Lancet*, **2**, 150
12. Daniell, H. W. (1973). Heparin in the prevention of infusion phlebitis. *J. Am. Med. Assoc.*, **225**, 1317

13. Editorial (1975). Venous thromboembolism and anticoagulants in pregnancy. *Br. Med. J.*, **4**, 421
14. Engelberg, H. (1975). The clinical use of heparin. *Curr. Ther. Res.*, **18**, 34
15. Eyer, K. M. (1973). Complications of transfemoral coronary arteriography and their prevention using heparin. *Am. Heart J.*, **85**, 428
16. Freid, M. O., Keave, J. F. and Rosenthall, A. (1974). The use of heparinization to prevent arterial thrombosis after percutaneous cardiac catheterization in children. *Circulation*, **90**, 565
17. Gardner, B. (1973). Experiences with the use of intracholedochal heparinized saline for the treatment of retained common duct stones. *Ann. Surg.*, **177**, 240
18. Hirsh, J., Cade, J. F. and Gallus, A. S. (1972). Anticoagulants in pregnancy: a review of indications and complications. *Am. Heart J.*, **83**, 301
19. McLean, J. (1916). The thromboplastic action of cephalin. *Am. J. Physiol.*, **41**, 250
20. Moore, F. D. (1973). Reflections on the new treatment for burns, caveat legor. *J. Am. Med. Assoc.*, **225**, 294
21. Saliba, M. J. (1968). Heparin in the treatment of burns. *J. Am. Med. Assoc.*, **200**, 650
22. Saliba, M. J. and Saliba, R. J. (1974). Heparin in burns: dose-related and dose-dependent effects. *Thromb. Diath. Haemorrh.*, **33**, 113
23. Sharnoff, J. G. Unpublished data
24. Touli, J., Jablonski, P. and Watts, J. M. (1975). Dissolution of human gallstones: the efficacy of bile salt, bile salt plus lecithin and heparin solution. *J. Surg. Res.*, **19**, 47

8

Prevention of Deep Vein Thrombosis and Pulmonary Embolism

Ever since Crafoord[15] recommended the use of postoperative intra-venous heparin in the prevention of thrombosis, many routines have been tried. The methods of prevention of deep vein thrombosis has had two main attacks based on two of the postulates of Virchow's original triad. The first attack was based on the assumption that slowing of the blood flow in the leg veins was the chief cause of deep vein thrombosis. This prompted the trial of early mobilization and ambulation following surgery. Then followed leg elevation, the wearing of elastic stockings[89], massage of the lower limbs, electrical stimulation of the calf muscles during surgery and the application of pneumatic boots[81] during surgery. These methods appeared to have had some beneficial effect in reducing the incidence of deep vein thrombosis but to a limited extent. Another method believed to improve blood flow was the use of the plasma expander dextran. More recently it has been shown that dextran[7,10,29,33] may also impair platelet aggregation and adhesiveness, an important cause of intravascular thrombosis. In addition, it has been described as a thrombolytic agent in the dissolution of already formed thrombi. Reports with the use of dextran 40 and 70 are contradictory, however. They also have adverse effects such as the overloading of the circulation and the necessity of repeated venous injections[29,30,82].

More recently, a number of more selective antiplatelet drugs have been tried. These include aspirin[11,16,32–34,36,42,43] dipyridamole[43], hydrochloroquine[91], sulphinpyrazone[10,11,16,32] and flurbiprofen[43]. There are many reports on the use of the above, often with contradictory results. All are in need of more extensive evaluation.

With the discovery of anticoagulants has also come the second attack on the most important of Virchow's postulates, namely, the prevention of intravascular coagulation or blood alteration referred to as hypercoagulation. The oral anticoagulants[33,58] were the first to be tried extensively. These included the dicourmarols and the phenindiones[58]. Although their dosage was controlled by prothrombin times and the more sophisticated partial thromboplastin times and activated plasma thromboplastin times, the severe haemorrhages they produced have resulted in the abandonment of their use in surgical procedures, There are still advocates for their use[33,58], with coumadin or warfarin and phenindione being the most popular. In the early years after its discovery heparin has been used to a limited degree to prevent thrombosis. Not until Jorpes in 1936 described its chemical structure and its action did Crafoord in 1937[15] report that heparin administered intravenously prophylactically in the postoperative period could prevent deep vein thrombosis. This was confirmed by deTakats in 1950[18], Bauer in 1954[5] and Lenggenhager in 1957[40] who administered smaller doses of intravenous heparin as suggested by deTakats[18]. In 1962 the author[68] advocated the use of (small dose) subcutaneous heparin sodium prophylactically preoperatively and postoperatively, but it was not until 1971[36] that the great wave of subcutaneous heparin anticoagulation research began. At the present time there are two chief programmes of subcutaneous heparin prophylaxis for the prevention of deep vein thrombosis and fatal pulmonary thromboembolism that have been tried extensively and proved to be effective. The first programme mentioned above is the monitored small dose regime developed by the author and the second is the fixed dose low dose regime. Trials with other antiplatelet substances such as aspirin and a combination of aspirin and other drugs such as dipyridamole, sulphinpyrazone and the above-mentioned are too few and contradictory for their efficacy to be convincing.

The monitored small dose regime was prompted by a series of human and animal studies described earlier[60-75] which indicated that the development of the hypercoagulable state and the likelihood of thrombosis was induced by the phenomenon of the pulmonary megakaryocytes. By anticipating hypercoagulation and employing an anticoagulant to prevent it, deep vein thrombosis and thromboembolism could both be avoided. When in 1957[60] the author observed that three patients who died of thrombotic thrombocytopenic purpura disclosed at autopsy a large number of megakaryocytes entrapped in the pulmonary precapillaries and capillaries, a series of studies to try to evaluate their significance was prompted. The cells known to be the source of platelet production in the bone marrow were first observed by Aschoff in the lung capillaries in 1893. He presumed that they had escaped intact from the bone marrow by the venous route, were carried to the lungs, and because of their giant size became entrapped in the lung capillaries. He described this as an end-stage, having no significance, an 'effete' phenomenon. The studies undertaken by the author and his colleagues[61,62,65] confirmed that these cells were truly megakaryocytes and that this was a normal process. The cells were found in all stages of fragmentation divided by the capillary anastomoses in humans and all mammals. With repeated right heart pulsations the cells emerged as fresh platelets in increased numbers in the heart's left ventricular blood and eventually in the peripheral blood producing a marked thrombocytosis. Often they were observed as giant platelets[64] having the configuration of casts of the pulmonary capillaries. When in 1959[63] the author observed that a marked increase in the number of megakaryocytes could be observed in the pulmonary capillaries of patients who had died from some form of thrombotic disease, it was postulated that this could be a priming effect. It was thought likely that any sudden increase in heart action, as with stress of any kind, would force the megakaryocytes through the pulmonary capillary anastomoses more rapidly.

This hypothesis was tested in rabbits by Sharnoff and Scardino[66] by sampling blood from the right and left ventricles. The study disclosed that there was no difference in platelet count in the blood from either heart ventricles. However, rabbits which were suddenly stressed while completely immobilized during a state of hibernation because of extreme winter cold, showed a marked increase in the number of platelets in the blood of the left heart ventricle. This increase was sometimes two to three times greater than the number found in the blood of the right heart ventricle. It was assumed that the hibernating immobilized animals had a lowered heart action, thereby slowing the forcing action on the capillary-entrapped megakaryocytes and thus the production of fresh platelets. The constant flow of megakaryocytes being released to the venous circulation meant their increasing entrapment in the pulmonary capillaries. This was considered the priming effect.

At this point an attempt was made to apply this concept to humans. Assuming that patients undergoing major elective surgery are subject to great stress, these could serve as experimental subjects[67]. Forty-one patients having major abdominal surgery had platelet counts and Lee–White coagulation times performed before, during and after surgery, with daily determinations made thereafter until discharge or death. There were three fatalities, all associated with a significant increase in platelets and shorter than normal coagulation times at the height of surgery. The remaining 38 patients had a less marked increase in platelets and normal though shorter coagulation times. Two of the three fatalities came to autopsy. One died suddenly of massive pulmonary thromboembolism on the second postoperative day. The second autopsied individual died on the twelfth postoperative day as a result of coronary artery thrombosis and an acute myocardial infarction which was estimated to have occurred on the day of surgery. Both were females 65 years of age who had undergone bowel resections for colonic carcinomas. The third fatal case was a 53-year-old male who had a subtotal gastrectomy for a benign peptic ulcer. He died suddenly from a clinically diagnosed massive pulmonary embolism when he was first allowed out of bed. Here, permission for autopsy was denied. The differences in coagulation times of the 38 who survived and the three who died of thrombosis or pulmonary embolism were significant. The survivors had normal coagulation times though revealing a shortened coagulation time at the peak of surgery, while the three fatal cases had shorter than normal coagulation times. Although these differences were small they prompted the concept that it would require small subcutaneous amounts of a predictable anticoagulant, easily controlled, to maintain normal levels of coagulation, thereby preventing thrombosis and avoiding haemorrhages. This meant maintaining a delicate balance between hypercoagulation and hypocoagulation.

Heparin sodium USP was chosen as the most likely anticoagulant to fulfil the need. This natural substance derived from the intestinal mucosa of the hog or bovine lung does not affect wound healing, has a limited predictable action, is easily neutralized by protamine sulphate, and is rarely affected by other medication, unlike the oral anticoagulants.

Beginning in August 1960[68], all operative patients of average size, having major, chiefly elective surgery, received 10 000 units of heparin sodium subcutaneously about midnight before the next morning's surgery. A baseline whole blood coagulation time preceded the injection. Following surgery, another whole blood coagulation time was determined and usually 2500 units of heparin were administered subcutaneously every 6 hours, depending on coagulation time values, until full remobilization or discharge. The coagulation time test was performed once daily before the next 12 noon administration of heparin. Small individuals under 50 kg were given 5000–7500 units of heparin about midnight before the next day's surgery and 2500 units every 6 hours postoperatively. Adjustment of postoperative heparin dosage depended on the coagulation times performed daily until discharge. The coagulation time was determined at the bedside by a simple reproducible whole blood test, using the Dale and Laidlaw coagulometer as modified by the author (described below). The test has a normal range of 1½ to 2½ minutes. The objective was to maintain blood coagulation in this range. Times shorter than 1½ minutes were deemed indicative of a hypercoagulable state and the test was repeated. If confirmed, the next dose of heparin was increased by 1000 units and this increased dose was continued every 6 hours until the next coagulation time and adjusted if necessary depending on the results obtained. Times longer than 2½ minutes were deemed indicative of hypocoagulation, and often one 6-hourly subcutaneous injection was omitted and the dose decreased by 1000 units and continued at the same dosage every 6 hours until the next before-noon coagulation time was determined. If necessary, the heparin dose was again adjusted as described above. When surgical patients are remobilized, especially following hip surgery or prolonged periods of immobilization, the modified Dale and Laidlaw coagulometer will usually indicate a markedly shortened coagulation time. This is a reflection of the sudden release of fresh platelets from the increased number of entrapped pulmonary megakaryocytes. This period must also be anticipated and the heparin dosage increased to neutralize the effect.

Author's (Small Dose) Heparin Regime

For patients having elective surgery

Step 1. Preoperative Dale and Laidlaw coagulometer time (control)

Step 2. Heparin sodium (porcine mucosal) USP at 12 midnight

Weight of patient	Dosage
100 lb (45 kg)	5000 units heparin subc.
Under 150 lb (68 kg)	7500 units heparin subc.
Over 150 lb (68 kg)	10 000 units heparin subc.
Over 200 lb (91 kg)	15 000 units heparin subc.

Step 3. Postoperative determination of coagulometer time in recovery room. (Normal range 1½–2½ minutes.) 2500 units heparin subc. every 6 hours – 6 am, 12 midday, 6 pm, 12 midnight.

Step 4. Daily coagulometer times before 12 noon. If shorter than 1½ minutes increase heparin by 1000 units every 6 hours. If prolonged more than 2½ minutes, decrease heparin by 1000 units every 6 hours.

Step 5. Continue heparinization until full ambulation and discharge of patient.

For patients having emergency hip fracture surgery

Step 1. As in Step 1 above immediately following admission until

surgery. 2500 units heparin every 6 hours.
Step 2.   Proceed as in Steps 2, 3, 4 and 5 above.

For medical patients (non-surgical)

As in Step 3 above until discharge.

Fixed Small Dose Heparin Regime

For elective thoracic and abdominal surgery only (not applicable to hip surgery)

Step 1.   5000 units of heparin calcium (or heparin sodium) subc. 2 hours before surgery. (Monitoring of heparin dosage not recommended.)
Step 2.   5000 units of heparin calcium subc. every 3–12 hours for 5–7 days postoperatively. (Monitoring or altering of heparin dosage not recommended.)

The fixed dose regime, on the other hand, first described in 1971[37], attempted to simplify subcutaneous heparin prophylaxis. This schedule called for a fixed heparin dose not requiring any monitoring test[38]. The authors advocated the subcutaneous administration of 5000 units of heparin 2 hours before surgery and the same dose every 8 hours for 5–7 days after operation. A monitoring test was deemed unnecessary because of the small amounts of heparin being administered and the finding that the usual control tests were not reliable[39]. However, it was soon determined that the fixed dose regime was not applicable to patients having hip surgery either elective or for hip fracture because of severe and at times fatal haemorrhages[12,24,25,41,43,46]. As a result, such patients were excluded from most studies including the large multicentre trial administered by Kakkar[44]. To quote Gallus and Engels, 'In contrast to its demonstrable value in elective intra-abdominal surgery, "low dose" heparin prophylaxis has little or no value in orthopaedic surgery'. They offered the explanation that patients undergoing hip surgery were of greater age and immobilized for long periods and may have already developed deep vein thrombosis before 'low dose' heparin prophylaxis was instituted for surgery. These assumptions are correct. Sevitt[58] recognized this in the use of prophylactic phenindione in patients having an operation for fractured hip and changed the schedule of prophylaxis accordingly. This was also observed by Galasko *et al.*[24]. About the same time the author[77] came to a similar conclusion independently and altered his (small dose) regime as administered to patients having acute hip surgery. He started preoperative heparin prophylaxis immediately following hospital admission. This was prompted from observations that patients with hip fractures requiring surgery, and having a loading dose of heparin the night before surgery, had the same incidence of fatal pulmonary embolism as patients not receiving any heparin prophylaxis. The incidence of fatal pulmonary embolism was 4.2% for the heparinized patients and 3.5% for those not receiving heparin. The failure in the heparinized group was presumed to be chiefly due to prolonged periods of immobilization (4–8 days) before surgery in four individuals. This prompted the change in the schedule to heparinize these patients as soon as possible following hospital admission. This meant administering heparin subcutaneously, usually 2500 units every 6 hours following admission until midnight before surgery when the usual loading dose was given. This was followed after operation with the 6-hourly schedule until the patient was remobilized and discharged. The results to date with this modified schedule have been very gratifying. In a series of over 250 patients with fractured hips there have not been any fatalities due to pulmonary embolism. This schedule also proved effective in avoiding severe haemorrhages, attributable to the fact that the author's (small dose) regime is carefully monitored and adjusted if necessary according to the response of each individual. Also, the simple, bedside modified Dale and Laidlaw coagulometer proved to be most reliable in maintaining normocoagulation.

The schedule of heparin prophylaxis for elective thoracic-abdominal surgical patients has also proved successful. By employing the loading dose schedule the night before surgery there has been only one postoperative fatality due to pulmonary thromboembolism. In a series of 3000 patients the single fatality might have been avoided if closer attention had been paid to that patient's hypercoagulable blood levels as determined by the modified Dale and Laidlaw coagulometer.

An altered schedule based upon the author's (small dose) regime of heparin prophylaxis has been applied to major elective abdominal surgery by DeBlasio (unpublished), monitored by the modified Dale and Laidlaw coagulometer. The DeBlasio regime consists of administering 5000 units of heparin sodium at 9.00 pm the night before surgery and 2000 units subcutaneously at 600 am on the day of surgery. After operation this schedule calls for 2000 units of heparin subcutaneously every 6 hours until discharge, and is altered if necessary according to coagulation times obtained with the coagulometer performed daily as described above. Haemorrhages of any severity have not been observed to date in several hundred patients treated as above. The DeBlasio regime is basically a fixed dose schedule for all patients regardless of body size. At times hypercoagulable blood levels have been observed with this schedule, and a rare clinically confirmed incidence of non-fatal pulmonary thromboembolism has been observed and treated successfully.

By contrast, the fixed (low dose) regime of subcutaneous heparin prophylaxis by recommending the omission of a heparin control accounts for the serious haemorrhages encountered with this regime and has caused many to abandon the method, not only in its use with thoracic-abdominal surgery, but also to completely exclude it with patients having hip surgery[12,17,24,41,47,48,84,85]. Another cause of serious haemorrhage is the timing of the fixed (low dose) heparin schedule. The latter recommends the subcutaneous administration of 5000 units of heparin 2 hours before major elective surgery followed by a similar dose every 8 hours and more recently every 12 hours for 5–7 days postoperatively. A heparin assay revealed that surgery was performed at the 'peak of heparin effect'[38]. This has been confirmed by Cooke[13], Nicolaides[47] and later the author[75] indicating that at 2–3 hours, surgery is being performed with hypocoagulable blood levels and readily explains the haemorrhages which have resulted. This has prompted some investigators[48,85] who have tried the fixed (low dose) regime to warn that this method can cause serious haemorrhages in some patients.

Deep vein thrombosis and pulmonary embolism appears to be another serious complication of the fixed (low dose) regime. The reason for this complication is that the programme recommends halting prophylaxis after 5–7 days. As a result this may induce deep vein thrombosis during a period when the patient is still immobilized and thus may not prevent the development of the second critical period of hypercoagulation, namely when the patient is remobilized, as observed by the author and colleagues[67]. The long period of immobilization that follows the period of prophylaxis, and the hypercoagulation on remobilization, may well produce deep vein thrombosis and the possibility of fatal or non-fatal pulmonary thromboembolism[76].

The discouraging results with the fixed (low dose) regime in hip surgery prompted the comment that the programme 'did not lend itself' to this form of surgery[38]. However, it is well known that hip surgery has the greatest incidence of fatal pulmonary thrombo-embolism and is in greatest need of this prophylaxis. However, the carefully monitored (small dose) heparin regime has been very effective in preventing fatal pulmonary embolism in hip cases as well[77].

Additional observations by the author indicate that it is essential to monitor heparin prophylaxis. Experience with the coagulometer has shown that the test is sensitive enough to indicate when errors of both omission and commission have been made in the administration of heparin. Patients receiving heparin prophylaxis who suddenly develop shorter than normal coagulation times will prove on investigation to have missed a dose. More often, prolonged coagulation times will on investigation disclose that an incorrectly large dose of heparin has been given or that an oral anticoagulant such as coumadin has been administered. The coagulometer is also capable of detecting the action of oral anticoagulants long before prothrombin times reflect it. Other drugs which can enhance the action of heparin such as papase, motrin (ibuprofen) and propranolol hydrochloride can also be reflected in the unusually prolonged coagulation times. Shortened coagulometer times may also be observed upon reactivation of a patient following a period of immobilization.

The difficulties encountered with the use of heparin reported by others have not been observed by the author during 18 years experience. It has been claimed that heparin is difficult to standardize[34] and that some patients are sensitive to the substance. It may well be that poor control tests, or the lack of them, may explain these difficulties. It has also been reported that a rebound effect may occur following the cessation of heparin therapy, but the author has not encountered this either.

As a result of the many reports that uncontrolled i.v. and fixed (low dose) heparin administrations have caused serious haemorrhages and deaths, a number of alternative methods of prophylaxis have been tried. Jaques et al.[35] recently proposed the inhalation of aerosol vapour of heparin, which produced a state of hypocoagulability lasting for days. The method remains to be evaluated.

Sagar et al.[56] have also proposed the use of calcium heparin as safer than sodium heparin in the prevention of serious haemorrhages especially in hip surgery. According to Berquist and Hallbrook[8] and Gruber et al.[30] their evaluation of calcium heparin indicates no significant difference in the anticoagulant effect of both heparins. This has also been confirmed by Nicolaides[47].

Thomas et al.[86] also attempting to reduce the incidence of haemorrhage with its fixed (low dose) regime, have tried a heparin analogue which potentiates antithrombin III *in vivo* while having little effect on overall clotting. This, too, remains to be evaluated.

More recently, the combination of antiplatelet drugs such as dipyridamole, sulphinpyrazone, hydrochloroquine and aspirin, or aspirin alone have been advocated. These are not fully evaluated yet and so far have had controversial reports. The chief advocates for aspirin appear to be Harris et al.[32] for orthopaedic surgery, chiefly hip surgery. Their reported material is small, besides indicating that aspirin is not an effective drug for females. Hume, commenting on the Harris report[34], indicated that his experience with aspirin prophylaxis in total hip replacement surgery, and administering a placebo as control, revealed no essential difference in the incidence of deep vein thrombosis. He failed to appreciate the observed sex difference in the Harris study.

Additional proposals by Browse et al.[10], and Smith et al.[82] recommended the use of dextran 70 in combination with pneumatic leg compression. They reported that dextran was more effective than intermittent leg compression, but that neither method alone prevented deep vein thrombosis. Smith et al.[82] reported postoperative bleeding and allergic reactions to dextran. Fatalities with the use of dextran have also been reported as a result of hypervolaemia.

Wessler[88] in the Lewis A. Connor Memorial Lecture in November 1976, at the American Heart Association meeting in Miami, presented an excellent summary of the present state of anticoagulant prophylaxis for the prevention of thromboembolism. He stated that although there was good evidence that heparin prophylaxis was effective in preventing pulmonary embolism it had not yet gained general acceptance in the United States or elsewhere. He referred to the use of subcutaneous heparin and the oral anticoagulants, estimating that this form of prophylaxis would prevent some 10 000 deaths annually in the United States alone (deaths in patients undergoing thoracic-abdominal surgery and those with acute myocardial infarctions). He also excluded their use in hip surgery where the need is generally recognized as greatest. Wessler made reference to the fixed (low dose) heparin prophylaxis regime generally administered without monitoring and the oral anticoagulant methods with poor control tests such as prothrombin times, partial thromboplastin times (PTT) and the activated partial thromboplastin time (APTT). Wessler is justified in his belief that the chief barrier to their use is the incidence of haemorrhages encountered with these methods. The lack of heparin and poor oral anticoagulant control account for the failure to use either of these methods of prophylaxis. This is especially true of the fixed (low dose) heparin regime because the above-mentioned monitoring methods lack the dependability, simplicity and immediacy required to determine the blood coagulation levels needed to adjust heparin dosage and so maintain the delicate balance between preventing thrombosis and avoiding haemorrhages.

Recently a controversy has arisen between participating members of the large multicentre trial which employed fixed (low dose) heparin prophylaxis for the prevention of thromboembolism. It appears that one participating institution[20] discovered that some of their patients with non-fatal as well as fatal thromboembolisms were not included in the final report to the *Lancet*[44]. This gave the reported results of the trial a more favourable outlook. When these facts came to light, Kakkar *et al.* of the multicentre study issued a reappraisal report[50] excluding all the cases of that centre[20] and claimed that the study still gave a highly significant result.

It is indeed difficult to understand this controversy, and Strandness[84] has recently voiced what many other investigators are thinking. The multicentre trial with fixed (low dose) heparin is the most extensive attempted to date and it is much to be regretted that the entire study has been questioned[84]. This has set back immeasurably a much needed programme of heparin prophylaxis and has probably caused a number of clinicians to abandon the fixed (low dose) regime which could well lead to unnecessary deaths.

It has been reported that heparin prophylaxis is ineffective in patients having prostatic surgery because excessive bleeding has been encountered in this type of surgery. Allen, Jenkins and Smart *et al.*[3] in a controlled study of 60 patients, 30 receiving the fixed (low dose) regime of calcium heparin and 30 not receiving any heparin, reported that six heparinized patients had haemorrhages requiring transfusion of two units of blood while the non-heparinized patients had no significant blood loss and did not require blood transfusion. Sharnoff and Rosenberg[70] in a retrospective review reported that following prostatectomies in men and hysterectomies in women there is a very low incidence of fatal pulmonary thromboembolism. It was also observed that the author's (small dose) heparin prophylaxis for prostatectomy is associated with increased blood loss compared to the non-heparinized prostatectomy patients. The blood loss is undoubtedly due to the inability to control bleeding sites in this procedure, and occurs to some degree without anticoagulation. It can be concluded that both the fixed (low dose) and the author's (small dose) regimes of heparin prophylaxis can prevent deep vein thrombosis and fatal pulmonary thromboembolism in the occasional prostatectomy patient, but tends to increase the amount of bleeding from the site of surgery.

The recommendation to be made is that if much morbidity and mortality is to be avoided, the heparin prophylaxis for the prevention of thromboembolism should be administered to all surgical patients at any adult age. This recommendation is made for all surgical and medical hospitalized patients who may be expected to be immobilized for any extended period of time.

Wallace and Evans[87] have made a significant observation. They have demonstrated that, costwise, routine preoperative and postoperative prophylaxis for the prevention of thromboembolism is far cheaper than screening for thrombosis or investigating for clinically suspected postoperative deep vein thrombosis and pulmonary embolism.

Thomas[85] has also commented succinctly, 'It is now necessary for physicians generally to recognize that as with all prophylactic therapy large numbers of patients must be treated to benefit the relatively few patients who would otherwise have suffered from thromboembolism'.

According to Rocko et al.[52], in an inquiry amongst United States general surgeons of their awareness of the prophylactic use of heparin sodium in small subcutaneous doses, 80% responded in the positive. But only 4% of surgical patients benefit from this form of prophylaxis. The reluctance on the part of surgeons to use heparin prophylaxis is the fear of haemorrhage from the fixed (low dose) regime[12,17,24,39,48,49,84,85] and their doubts about the laboratory monitoring generally employed.

It is clear from the evidence presented that in the forseeable future it is advisable for the author's carefully monitored, safe (small dose) regime of heparin prophylaxis to be the method against which all other prophylactic methods for the prevention of thromboembolism are measured. It is an urgent necessity for such a regime to be adopted as a routine hospital procedure if the morbidity and mortality of this common, ever-increasing problem is to be prevented.

References

1. Abernethy, E. E. and Hartsuck, J. M. (1974). Postoperative pulmonary embolism. A prospective study utilizing low-dose heparin. *Am. J. Surg.*, **128**, 739
2. Abdou-Abdallah, E., Rausis, C., Loup, P. and Mosimann, R. (1975). Etude comparative heparinate de sodium et de calcium dans la prophylazie des maladies thrombo-emboliques en chirurgie. *Helv. Chir. Acta*, **42**, 691
3. Allen, N. H., Jenkins, J. D. and Smart, C. J. (1978). Surgical haemorrhage in patients given subcutaneous heparin as prophylaxis against thrombo-embolism. *Br. Med. J.*, **1**, 326
4. Baskin, H. E., Murray, J. M. and Harris, R. E. (1977). Low-dose heparin for prevention of thromboembolic disease in pregnancy. *Am. J. Obstet. Gynecol.*, **129**, 590
5. Bauer, G. (1954). Thirteen years experience with heparin therapy. In Koller, T. and Merz, W. (eds.). *Proceedings of the 1st Conference on Thrombosis and Embolism*, Basel, p. 721
6. Bauer, G. (1955). Prophylaxis and therapy of thrombosis of legs. *Nord. Med.*, **53**, 779
7. Bergentz, S. E. (1978). Dextran in prophylaxis of pulmonary embolism. *World J. Surg.*, **2**, 19
8. Berquist, D. and Hallbrook, T. (1977). Are there any differences in thrombosis, prophylaxis and the side effects between sodium and calcium heparin? *Proceedings of the 6th International Congress on Thrombosis and Hemostasis*, p. 106
9. Bern, M. M. (1975). Variable response of activated partial thromboplastin time in heparin therapy during hemodialysis. *Am. J. Clin. Pathol.*, **64**, 602
10. Browse, N. L., Clemenson, G., Bateman, N. T., Gaunt, J. I. and Croft, D. N. (1976). Effect of intravenous dextran 70 and pneumatic leg compression on incidence of postoperative pulmonary embolism. *Br. Med. J.*, **2**, 1281
11. Canadian Cooperative Study Group (1978). A randomized trial of aspirin and sulfinpyrazone in threatened stroke. *N. Engl. J. Med.*, **299**, 53
12. Charnley, J. (1972). Prophylaxis of postoperative thromboembolism. *Lancet*, **2**, 134

13. Cooke, E. D., Lloyd, M. J., Bowcock, S. A. and Pilcher, M. F. (1976). Monitoring during low-dose heparin prophylaxis. *N. Engl. J. Med.*, **294**, 1066

14. Council on Thrombosis of the American Heart Association (1977). Prevention of venous thromboembolism in surgical patients by low dose heparin. *Circulation*, **55**, 423A

15. Crafoord, C, (1936). Preliminary report on post-operative treatment with heparin as a preventative of thrombosis. *Acta Chir. Scand.*, **77**, 407

16. Dechavanne, M., Ville, D., Viala, J. J., Kher, A., Faivre, J., Pousset, M. B. and Dejour, H. (1975). Controlled trial of platelet anti-aggregating agents and subcutaneous heparin in prevention of postoperative deep vein thrombosis in high risk patients. *Hemostasis*, **4**, 94

17. Dechavanne, M., Soudin, F., Viala, J. J., Kher, A., Bertrix, L. and deMourgues, G. (1974). Prevention des thromboses veineuses. Succès de l'heparin a fortes doses des coxarthroses. *Nouv. Presse Med.*, **3**, 1317

18. deTakats, G. (1950). Anticoagulation in surgery. *J. Am. Med. Assoc.*, **142**, 507

19. deTakats, G. (1977). Small-dose prophylactic heparin. *Mod. Med.*, Oct., 38

20. Duckert, F., Gruber, U. F., Fridrich, R., Torhorst, J. and Rem, J. (1977). Low-dose heparin. *Lancet*, **2**, 1163

21. Editorial (1975). Low-dose heparin and the prevention of venous thromboembolic disease. *Br. Med. J.*, **2**, 447

22. Editorial (1975). Prevention of fatal post-operative pulmonary embolism by low doses of heparin. *Lancet*, **1**, 145

23. Freiman, D. G., Syemoto, J. and Wessler, S. (1965). Frequency of pulmonary thromboembolism in man. *N. Engl. J. Med.*, **272**, 1278

24. Galasko, C. S., Edwards, D. H., Fearn, C. B. D. and Barker, H. M. (1976). The value of low dosage heparin for the prophylaxis of thromboembolism in patients with transcervical and intertrochanteric femoral fractures. *Acta Orthop. Scand.*, **47**, 276

25. Gallus, A. S., Hirsh, J., Tuttle, R. J., Trebilcock, R., O'Brien, S. E., Carroll, J. J., Minden, J. H. and Hudecki, S. M. (1973). Small subcutaneous doses of heparin in prevention of venous thrombosis. *N. Engl. J. Med.*, **288**, 545

26. Gallus, A. S., Hirsh, J., O'Brien, S. E., McBride, J. A., Tuttle, R. J. and Gent, M. (1976). Prevention of venous thrombosis with small subcutaneous doses of heparin. *J. Am. Med. Assoc.*, **235**, 1980

27. Gordon-Smith, I. C., Grundy, D. J., LeQuesne, L. P. and Newcombe, J. F. (1972). Controlled trial of two regimens of subcutaneous heparin in prevention of post-operative deep vein thrombosis. *Lancet*, **1**, 1132

28. Gordon-Smith, I. C., LeQuesne, L. P. and Newcombe, J. F. (1974). Subcutaneous heparin and postoperative venous thrombosis. *Lancet*, **2**, 286

29. Gruber, U. F., Duckert, F., Fridrich, R., Torhorst, J. and Rem, J. (1977). Prevention of postoperative thromboembolism by ·dextran 40, low doses of heparin or xantinol nicotinate. *Lancet*, **1**, 207

30. Gruber, U. F., Rem, J., Altorfer, R., Schaub, N., Freddie, K. E., Fridrich, R. and Duckert, F. (1973). Efficacy of dextran 40 or heparin in prevention of deep vein thrombosis after major surgery. *Eur. Surg. Res.* (Suppl. 2), **5**, 15

31. Harris, W. H. (1976). Low-dose heparin in total hip replacement. *Lancet*, **2**, 423

32. Harris, W. A., Salzman, E. W., Athanasoulis, C. A., Waltman, A. C., and DeSanctis, R. W. (1977). Aspirin prophylaxis of venous thromboembolism after total hip replacement. *N. Engl. J. Med.*, **297**, 1246

33. Harris, W. H., Salzman, E. W., Athanasoulis, C. A., Waltman, A. C., Baum, S. and DeSanctis, R. W. (1974). Comparison of warfarin, low-molecular weight dextran, aspirin, and subcutaneous heparin in prevention of venous thromboembolism following total hip replacement. *J. Bone Jt. Surg.*, **56A**, 1552

34. Hume, M. (1978). Aspirin for prophylaxis of venous thromboembolism. *N. Engl. J. Med.*, **298**, 1091

35. Jaques, L. B., Mahados, J. and Kavanaugh, L. W. (1976). Intrapulmonary heparin. *Lancet*, **2**, 1157

36. Jennings, J. J., Harris, W. H. and Sarmiento, A. (1976). A clinical evaluation of aspirin prophylaxis after total hip arthroplasty. *J. Bone Jt. Surg.*, **58A**, 926

37. Kakkar, V. V., Field, E. S., Nicolaides, A. N., Flute, P. T., Wessler, S. and Yin, E. T. (1971). Low doses of heparin in the prevention of deep vein thrombosis. *Lancet*, **2**, 669

38. Kakkar, V. V., Corrigan, T. P., Spindler, J., Fossard, D. P., Flute, P. T., Crellin, R. Q., Wessler, S. and Yin, E. T. (1972). Efficacy of low doses of heparin in prevention of deep vein thrombosis after major surgery. A double blind randomized trial. *Lancet*, **2**, 101

39. Kakkar, V. V. (1978). The current status of low-dose heparin prophylaxis of thrombophlebitis and pulmonary embolism. *World J. Surg.*, **2**, 3

40. Lenggenhager, K. (1957). Genese und prophylaxes der postoperatiren fernthrombose. *Helv. Chir. Acta*, **24**, 316

41. Mannucci, P. M., Citterio, L. E. and Panjotopoulous, N. (1976). Low-dose heparin and deep vein thrombosis after total hip replacement. *Thromb. Hemostas.*, **36**, 167

42. Medical Research Council (1972). Effect of aspirin on postoperative venous thrombosis. *Lancet*, **2**, 441

43. Morris, G. K. and Mitchell, J. R. A. (1977). Preventing venous thromboembolism in elderly patients with hip fractures: studies of low dose heparin, dipyridamole, aspirin and flurbiprofen. *Br. Med. J.*, **1**, 535

44. Multicentre Trial (1975). Prevention of fatal postoperative pulmonary embolism by low doses of heparin. *Lancet*, **2**, 45

45. Nicolaides, A. N., Dupont, P. A., Desai, S., Lewis, J. D., Douglas, J. N., Dodsworth, H., Fourides, G., Luck, R. J. and Jamieson, C. W. (1972). Small doses of subcutaneous sodium heparin in preventing deep venous thrombosis after major surgery. *Lancet*, **2**, 890

46. Nicolaides, A. N., Dupont, P., Parsons, D., Appleberg, M., Horan, F. T., Esah, K. M. and Walker, C. J. (1974). Small dose subcutaneous sodium heparin in preventing deep venous thrombosis after elective hip surgery. *Br. J. Surg.*, **61**, 320

47. Nicolaides, A. N. (1978). Invited commentary to V. V. Kakkar – Heparin prophylaxis of thromboembolism. *World J. Surg.*, **2**, 13

48. Pachter, H. L. and Riles, T. S. (1977). Low dose heparin: bleeding and wound complications in the surgical patient, a prospective randomized study. *Ann. Surg.*, **186**, 669

49. Poller, L., Thomson, J. M. and Yee, K. F. (1977). Stability studies on lyophilized reference thromboplastins for standardization of prothrombin times. *Lancet*, **2**, 1019

50. Reappraisal of results of international multicentre trial. Prevention of fatal postoperative pulmonary embolism by low doses of heparin. (1977). *Lancet*, **1**, 567

51. Roberts, V. C. and Cotter, L. T. (1975). Failure of low dose heparin to improve efficacy of preoperative intermittent calf compression in preventing deep vein thrombosis. *Br. Med. J.*, **3**, 458

52. Rocko, J. M., Mikhail, F., Trilles, F. and Timmes, J. J. (1978). The safety of low dose heparin prophylaxis. *Am. J. Surg.*, **135**, 798

53. Rosenberg, R. D. (1974). Heparin action. *Circulation*, **49**, 603

54. Rubin, R. N. (1978). Aspirin and post surgery bleeding. *Ann. Intern. Med.*, **89**, 1006

55. Sagar, S., Massey, J. and Sanderson, J. M. (1975). Low dose heparin prophylaxis against fatal pulmonary embolism. *Br. Med. J.*, **4**, 257

56. Sagar, S., Nairn, D., Stamatakis, J. D., Maffei, F. H., Higgins, A. F., Thomas, D. P. and Kakkar, V. V. (1976). Efficacy of low-dose heparin in prevention of extensive deep vein thrombosis in patients undergoing total hip replacement. *Lancet*, **1**, 1151

57. Salzman, E. W., Deykin, D., Shapiro, R. M. and Rosenberg, R. (1975). Management of heparin therapy controlled prospective study. *New. Engl. J. Med.*, **292**, 1046

58. Sevitt, S. and Gallager, N. G. (1959). Prevention of venous thrombosis and pulmonary embolism in injured patients. *Lancet*, **2**, 981

59. Sevitt, S. (1970). In Hume, M., Sevitt, S. and Thomas, D. P. (eds.). *Venous Thrombosis and Pulmonary Embolism*, p. 380. (Cambridge: Harvard University Press)

60. Sharnoff, J. G. (1957). Thrombotic thrombocytopenic purpura. *Am. J. Med.*, **23**, 740

61. Sharnoff, J. G., and Kim, E. S. (1958). Evaluation of pulmonary megakaryocytes. *Arch. Pathol.*, **66**, 176

62. Sharnoff, J. G. and Kim, E. S. (1958). Pulmonary megakaryocyte studies in rabbits. *Arch. Pathol.*, **66**, 340

63. Sharnoff, J. G., (1959). Increased pulmonary megakaryocytes – probable role in postoperative thromboembolism. *J. Am. Med. Assoc.*, **169**, 688

64. Sharnoff, J. G. (1959). A possible explanation of the formation of long platelets from pulmonary megakaryocytes. *Nature (London)*, **184**, 75

65. Sharnoff, J. G. and Scardino, V. (1959). Pulmonary megakaryocytes in human fetuses and premature and full-term infants. *Arch. Pathol.*, **69**, 139

66. Sharnoff, J. G. and Scardino, V. (1960). Platelet count differences in blood of rabbit right and left heart ventricles. *Nature (London)*, **187**, 334

67. Sharnoff, J. G., Bagg, J. F., Breen, S. R., Rogliano, A. G., Walsh, A. R. and Scardino, V. (1960). The possible indication of postoperative thromboembolism by platelet counts and blood coagulation studies in the patient undergoing extensive surgery. *Surg. Gynecol. Obstet.*, **111**, 469

68. Sharnoff, J. G., Kass, H. H. and Mistica, B. A. (1962). A plan of heparin-

ization of the surgical patient to prevent postoperative thromboembolism. *Surg. Gynecol. Obstet.*, **115**, 75

69. Sharnoff, J. G. (1963). An evaluation of the Dale and Laidlaw coagulometer in the heparin control of thromboembolism. *Proc. NY State Assoc. Pub. Hlth. Labs.*, **43**, 10

70. Sharnoff, J. G. and Rosenberg, M. (1964). Effects of age and immobilization on the incidence of postoperative thromboembolism. *Lancet*, **1**, 845

71. Sharnoff, J. G. (1966). Results in the prophylaxis of postoperative thromboembolism. *Surg. Gynecol. Obstet.*, **123**, 303

72. Sharnoff, J. G. (1966). Post mortem findings in 25 cases of sudden heart arrest in the perioperative period. *Lancet*, **2**, 876

73. Sharnoff, J. G. (1969). Prevention of sudden cardio-pulmonary arrest in the perioperative period with prophylactic heparin. *Lancet*, **2**, 292

74. Sharnoff, J. G. and DeBlasio, G. (1970). Prevention of fatal post-operative thromboembolism by heparin prophylaxis. *Lancet*, **2**, 1006

75. Sharnoff, J. G. and DeBlasio, G. (1970). Some implications in the successful heparin prophylaxis of sudden cardio-pulmonary arrest by thrombosis and embolism. *Am. Heart J.*, **80**, 848

76. Sharnoff, J. G. (1973). Prevention of thromboembolism. *Bull NY Acad. Med.*, **49**, 655

77. Sharnoff, J. G., Rosen, R. L., Sadler, A. H. and Ibarra-Isunza, G. C. (1976). Prevention of pulmonary thromboembolism by heparin prophylaxis after surgery for hip fractures. *J. Bone Jt. Surg.*, **58A**, 913

78. Sharnoff, J. G. (1975). Prevention of postoperative thromboembolism. *Lancet*, **2**, 361

79. Sharnoff, J. G. (1977). Low dose or small dose heparin. *Lancet*, **2**, 1087

80. Sherry, S. (1975). Low-dose heparin prophylaxis for postoperative venous thromboembolism. *N. Engl. J. Med.*, **273**, 300

81. Skillman, J. J., Collins, R. E., Coe, N. P., Goldstein, B. S., Shapiro, R. M., Zervas, N. T., Bettman, M. A. and Salzman, E. W. (1978). Prevention of deep vein thrombosis in neurosurgical patients: a controlled randomized trial of external pneumatic compression boots. *Surgery*, **83**, 354

82. Smith, R. C., Elton, P. A., Orr, J. D., Hart, A. J. L., Graham, D. F., Fuller, G. A. G., Rundle, J. S. H., McPherson, A. I. S. and Ruckley, C. V. (1978). Dextran and intermittent pneumatic compression in prevention of deep vein thrombosis: multicentre trial. *Br. Med. J.*, **1**, 1031

83. Stamatakis, J. D., Kakkar, V. V., Lawrence, D., Bentley, P. G., Nairn, D. and Ward, V. (1978). Failure of aspirin to prevent post-operative deep vein thrombosis in patients undergoing total hip replacement. *Br. Med. J.*, **1**, 1031

84. Strandness, D. E. Jr. (1978). Invited commentary to Kakkar, V. V. – Heparin prophylaxis of thromboembolism. *World J. Surg.*, **2**, 17

85. Thomas, D. P. (1978). Heparin in prophylaxis and treatment of venous thromboembolism. *Semin. Hematol.*, **15**, 1

86. Thomas, D. P., Lane, D. A., Michalski, P., Johnson, E. M. and Kakkar, V. V. (1977). A heparin analogue with specific action on antithrombin III. *Lancet*, **1**, 120

87. Wallace, W. A. and Evans, C. M. (1976). Venous thromboembolism: a cost

evaluation of prophylaxis, investigation and treatment. *J. R. Coll. Surg. Edinburgh*, **2**, 218

88. Wessler, S. (1977). The anticoagulant dilemma – a prescription for its resolution. *Am. J. Med. Sci.*, **274**, 107
89. Wilkens, R. W., Mixter, Jr. G., Stanton, J. R. and Litter, J. (1952). Elastic stockings in the prevention of pulmonary embolism: a preliminary report. *N. Engl. J. Med.*, **246**, 360
90. Williams, H. T. (1971). Prevention of postoperative deep vein thrombosis with perioperative subcutaneous heparin. *Lancet*, **2**, 950
91. Chrisman, O. D., Snook, E. A., Wilson, T. C. and Short, J. Y. (1976). Prevention of venous thrombo bolism by administration of hydrochloroquine. A preliminary report. *J. Bone Jt. Surg.*, **58**, 918

9

Diagnosis of Deep Vein Thrombosis and Pulmonary Thromboembolism

The clinical diagnosis of the presence of deep vein thrombosis and pulmonary thromboembolism has always been unreliable[41], particularly with regard to physical signs and symptoms. The latter are the well known Homan's sign, pain and tenderness in the calf muscles, swelling and palpation of cords in the leg and thigh muscles, and skin discoloration (cyanosis). Objective techniques have shown that the clinical physical signs are only 50% or less accurate, with a frequent false-positive diagnosis.

The newer objective techniques for the diagnosis of deep vein thrombosis may be divided into the invasive and non-invasive methods[3,26]. The invasive methods most commonly used are venography[9,15,19,31,32,36,45,52,55,64,65] and the [^{125}I]fibrinogen test. Venography, despite its drawbacks such as incomplete filling of vein lumens and muscle compression of the vessels, still has a 90% accuracy so it is perhaps the most reliable method of detecting deep vein thrombosis. When venography is negative it is considered 100% reliable. To avoid the above-mentioned drawbacks, the modified method of Rabinov and Paulin[54] is generally used.

With the patient on an X-ray table tilted at 40° and the legs lowered, a radio-opaque solution of about 150 ml is injected into a vein of the dorsum of the foot, under fluoroscopic control. The legs must be kept fully relaxed. Spot X-ray films are obtained in both anterior–posterior and lateral projection during venous filling. Overhead radiographs including films over the pelvic area are also obtained. Following this procedure the patient is returned to the flat position and the veins are flushed with 150 ml of an isotonic solution of 2500 units of heparin sodium. This should be done immediately since contrast medium is irritating to the venous intima, so there may be the risk of thrombosis.

The [125I]fibrinogen test[7,10,13,23,25,31,35,39], the second most commonly used invasive method, depends on the intravenous injection of [125I]fibrinogen. This is incorporated in a developing thrombus which becomes radioactive and can be detected with a scintillation counter. The test, however, has its dangers and limitations; difficulties can be encountered in elderly patients[27] following the administration of potassium iodide which is usually administered 24 hours before the [125I]fibrinogen is given to prevent the thyroid from absorbing the free 125I. The test can be used in two ways; in the anticipation of leg vein thrombosis in high risk patients, or to demonstrate the presence of thrombi. Until recently the United States Food and Drug Administration prohibited its use owing to the risk of Australia antigen in the fibrinogen and the danger of hepatitis. The method should not be used in pregnant or nursing women as it cannot detect thrombi in the pelvic area[24,27,29,39,42,44].

Sodium iodide may also be used to minimize the thyroid uptake of radioiodine. This is continued for 2–3 weeks. A single injection of [125I]fibrinogen allows for leg scanning of 8–10 days. The patient's legs are elevated to 30–40° to prevent pooling in the leg veins. The radioactivity is expressed as a percentage. Venous thrombosis is diagnosed if there is an increase in the value of the percentage radioactivity by 20 at any point, provided this persists for 24 hours or longer.

There are several serious limitations to the [125I]fibrinogen test. It is completely insensitive to pelvic vein thrombosis and quite inaccurate in the proximal one-third of the thigh. Extravascular fibrinogen uptake occurs in infected wounds, haematomas or healing wounds. As a result it is most limited in orthopaedic or leg surgery. Background radioactivity from the bladder interferes with the accuracy of the test. However, both venography and [125I]fibrinogen leg scanning are basically research tools, costly, painful, time-consuming, involving special equipment and trained staff; they can, however, serve to confirm the efficacy of prophylactic measures, so when these become widely used it would eliminate the need for such techniques including the non-invasive methods.

Among the more commonly used non-invasive methods for the demonstration of deep vein thrombosis are the Doppler ultrasound flowmeter method[7,22,28,34,61,62,68], impedance plethysmography[9,16,18,20], and thermography[14]. With ultrasound venous flow or its absence is detected audibly. As a diagnostic method for the determination of clinically suspected deep vein thrombosis it has been investigated extensively. It has been shown to be highly sensitive in popliteal, femoral and iliac vein thrombosis, but of low sensitivity in calf vein thrombosis. However, Barnes et al.[5] have also reported good results in the latter. As a test for deep vein thrombosis it compares very favourably with the invasive methods especially venography[33].

The test is simple to perform and results are obtained rapidly. Experience is essential for the proper interpretation of the findings. The examination is carried out with the patient lying relaxed in bed and the head slightly raised. The Doppler ultrasound velocity detector is a portable hand-held probe with transmission frequency of 5 MHz. It contains an oscillator which activates a piezoelectric crystal so that it emits an ultrasound beam; the frequency of the emitted beam is reflected percutaneously from blood cells in an underlying vein. The flow velocity signal in the vein is low pitched, and is affected by respiration and distinct from arterial blood flow. The flow velocity signals of the common femoral, superficial femoral, popliteal veins are examined in turn, and the spontaneity, augmentation and competence of the signals is noted at each location. The presence of thrombosis in the deep veins is characterized by the absence of venous flow signal, or by loss of velocity fluctuation with respiration, or augmentation of velocity in response to compression of the distal part of the limb or a Valsalva manoeuvre. It is often helpful if a comparison can be made with flow studies on the opposite limb if normal. For a more detailed description of technique the reader is referred to Barnes et al.[6]

Impedance plethysmography on the other hand is based on the

observation that changes in the calf blood volume as produced by maximum respiratory effort, or by inflation and deflation of a pneumatic thigh cuff, result in changes of electrical resistance. There are many reports in the literature describing the test in greater detail; the test is now performed as occlusive impedance plethysmography. The patient is supine with the lower extremity elevated; a midthigh pneumatic cuff is inflated to occlude venous return flow and after a period of time the cuff is rapidly deflated. The changes of electrical impedance during inflation and deflation are traced on a recorder, with the tracing rising on cuff inflation and falling after deflation. In this way normal and abnormal graphs are clearly differentiated. Often both the above non-invasive methods are employed for greater accuracy of diagnosis for deep vein thrombosis.

Another non-invasive method worthy of mention in the diagnosis of deep vein thrombosis is thermography. It is still in limited use because it is costly and has the additional drawback, as with the other non-invasive techniques, of not being objective. Here infrared photography is employed to determine the presence of vein thrombosis by recording the slight difference in temperature over the areas of thrombosis. As suggested by Cooke and Pilcher[14,29], projecting the image on a screen improves the chances of correct interpretation of the films. More recently a new non-invasive technique was suggested for the diagnosis of deep vein thrombosis by Simon and Krakenbuhl[59] based upon the principle of venous stop-flow pressure measurement. As yet not evaluated by others, it measures the pressure (as recorded by patients inhaling into a water manometer) that is necessary to stop the flow of blood in the deep veins of the legs. Apparently greater pressures are required when deep vein thrombosis is present.

Blood tests have also been devised in an attempt to determine the presence of deep vein thrombosis[33]. The staphylococcal clumping test is perhaps the most reliable. Here fibrin-split products indicate the presence of a thrombus which is in the process of dissolving. It has rather limited usefulness as, for instance, it cannot distinguish between thromboses and blood clots in the wounds of recently operated patients. Here again prophylaxis will limit its use. In the presence of thrombosis, however, the test can be of help.

The diagnosis of pulmonary embolism is often also very inaccurate[56] both clinically and radiographically. The most common clinical signs are dramatic, sudden collapse, air hunger, cyanosis, and shock. Less common are pleuritic chest pain, apprehension, cough, haemoptysis, syncope and substernal chest pain in that order of frequency. It is often a medical catastrophe and frequently the most rapid death known to man.

Should the patient survive for a longer period before radiographic confirmation can be obtained it is often too late to initiate lifesaving surgery. In addition, it may well be that the patient would have survived without surgical intervention, for it is true that pulmonary thromboembolism with or without infarction of the lung occurs far more frequently without a fatal outcome than is commonly believed. Radiographically, two methods are in common use to confirm the diagnosis: the perfusion lung scan and the pulmonary angiogram, in addition to the plain chest film. With the latter, less than 50% will reveal pulmonary consolidation and high diaphragms. Still fewer will reveal pleural effusions and atelectasis.

Perfusion lung scanning[8,10,15,25,26,31,42,56,63,65] is carried out by the venous injection of macroaggregated albumin tagged with ^{99m}Tc with the aggregates small enough to enter the pulmonary capillaries. The half-life of ^{99m}Tc is about 6 hours – long enough to carry out definitive studies. The method is relatively simple and safe needing only a proper electronic scanning device. Multiple projections are necessary for proper evaluation, although the smallest emboli may not be detected by this method. It is far more reliable than other techniques, especially compared to angiography, and should be the method of choice.

Angiography is more difficult to perform. It should be carried out by catheterization and instillation of Renografin 76. The site of investigation should be selective depending on clinically and radiographically suspicious areas of involvement. Occlusion of the larger vessels is readily visualized. Among conditions which may cause failures with this method are inflammatory disease, venous obstruction such as tumours, local thrombosis, chest masses, aneurysms, bronchial cysts, bullous emphysema and atelectasis. In addition there are hazards: fatalities with this method have been reported and temporary hypotension may occur; perforation of the right ventricle is rare. It is essential to monitor by ECG during angiography.

The plain chest film should be obtained before attempting the scan or angiography. Here decreased vascular markings are most significant in the presence of suspicious clinical symptoms, especially shock and air hunger. Absent or decreased vascular markings are usually associated with greater radiolucency of the involved areas. However this will be present in less than 50% of cases. Often the film will appear normal in the presence of embolism. Most often pulmonary thromboembolism is bilateral, limiting the value of the plain film since a comparison cannot be made with both lung areas.

Pulmonary infarction may be recognized on the plain film. It is, however, an infrequent accompaniment of embolism. Far fewer infarcts than 10% are noted at autopsy in the presence of an embolism. This is perhaps due to the fact that death through embolism occurs with such rapidity that infarction fails to develop. When recognized on the plain film it may represent an earlier embolism and not a new development. The X-ray findings of infarction, namely a radio-opaque zone as a triangular area with its base on the pleural surface and the apex pointing towards the hilum of the lung, are classic. Multiple infarcts are frequent and may occur sequentially. They may take a few hours to form and remain visible for at least a week or a few weeks. Often infarcts may not have the classic appearance as described above.

Still less reliable indications for the diagnosis of pulmonary embolism are the ECG changes suggestive of right-sided hypertension, or the biochemical changes that appear as sudden increases in enzymes such as alkaline phosphatase or serum lactic acid dehydrogenase. The ECG may help in differentiating pulmonary embolism from acute myocardial infarction.

It should be emphasized that prevention of thromboembolism has greater priority but should it occur independently despite prophylaxis then therapy becomes vital. This will be discussed below. In most instances, however, should the patient survive, the emboli or the infarcts will resolve spontaneously. The emboli will become adherent to the blood vessel wall and through endotheliazation will become organized and recanalized. The pulmonary infarct, which consists of blood filling the alveolar sacs, will cause necrosis of the infarcted area of the lung, and also absorb, organize and lead to scar formation often difficult to recognize. This condition may take weeks to develop.

Other new and as yet not fully evaluated invasive methods of diagnosis of deep vein thrombosis include isotope-labelled urokinase[51], streptokinase[21], plasmin[32,36] and leukocytes[12]. Much more experience is needed to assess the above methods.

More recently a rheographic, non-invasive method of diagnosis of deep vein thrombosis has been devised. In essence it is a plethysmographic method which measures hydraulic changes. It has been highly recommended by Cranley et al.[17]. Simon and Krakenbuhl[59] also recommend a venous stop-flow pressure method for diagnosing deep vein thrombosis. These also remain to be evaluated further by other centres.

References

1. Albrechtson, V. and Olsson, C. G. (1976). Thrombotic side-effects of lower limb phlebography. *Lancet*, **1**, 723
2. Athanasoulis, C. A. (1975). Phlebography for the diagnosis of deep leg vein thrombosis. *National Institute of Health DHEW* Publication No. 76–866, p. 62
3. Atkins, P. and Hawkins, L. A. (1965). Detection of venous thrombosis in the legs. *Lancet*, **2**, 1217
4. Barnes, R. W., Collicott, P. I., Mozersky, D., Sumner, D. S. and Strandness, D. E. Jr. (1972). Non-invasive quantitation of maximum venous outflow in acute thrombophlebitis. *Surgery*, **72**, 971
5. Barnes, R. W., Russell, H. E., Wm, K. K. and Hoats, J. C. (1976). Accuracy of Doppler ultrasound in clinically suspected venous thrombosis of the calf. *Surg. Gynecol. Obstet.*, **43**, 425
6. Barnes, R. W., Russell, H.E. and Wilson, M.R. (1975). *Doppler Ultrasonic Evaluation of Venous Disease. A Programmed Audio-visual Instruction.* 2nd Edition. (Iowa City: University of Iowa Press)
7. Becker, J. (1972). The diagnosis of venous thrombosis in the legs using I-labelled fibrinogen, an experimental and clinical study. *Acta Chir. Scand.*, **138**, 667
8. Bell, W. R. (1975). The diagnosis of pulmonary embolism: a comparison between lung perfusion scans and pulmonary angiograms. *National Institute of Health DHEW* Publication No. 76–866, p. 113
9. Berquist, E., Berquist, D., Bronge, A., Dahlgren, S. and Hallbrook, T. (1973). Diagnosis of venous thrombosis in the lower limbs: a comparative study between ^{125}I fibrinogen test, strain gauge plethysmography and phlebography. *UPS J. Med. Sci.*, **78**, 191
10. Browse, N. L., Clemenson, G. and Croft, D. N. (1974). Fibrinogen detectable thrombosis in the legs and pulmonary embolism. *Br. Med. J.*, **1**, 603
11. Bynum, L. J. and Wilson, J. E. (1978). Phleborheography for thrombosis. *Ann. Intern. Med.*, **89**, 1006
12. Charkes, N. D., Dugan, M. A., Malmud, L. S., Stern, H., Anderson, H.,

Kozan, J. and Maguire, R. (1974). Labelled leucocytes in thrombi. *Lancet*, **2**, 600

13. Coleman, R. E., Krohn, K. R., Metzger, J. M., Welch, M. J., Sacker-Walker, R. H. and Siegel, B. A. (1974). An *in vivo* evaluation of I-fibrinogen labelled by four different methods. *J. Lab. Clin. Med.*, **83**, 972

14. Cooke, E. D. and Pilcher, M. F. (1974). Deep vein thrombosis, preclinical diagnosis by thermography. *Br. J. Surg.*, **61**, 971

15. Corrigan, J. P., Fossard, D. P., Spindler, J., Armstrong, P., Strachan, C. J. L., Johnston, K. W. and Kakkar, V. V. (1974). Phlebography in the management of pulmonary embolism. *Br. J. Surg.*, **61**, 484

16. Cranley, J. J., Gay, A. Y., Grass, A. M. and Simeone, F. A. (1973). A plethysmographic technique for the diagnosis of deep vein thrombosis of the lower extremities. *Surg. Gynecol. Obstet.*, **136**, 385

17. Cranley, J. J., Canos, A. J., Sull, W. J. and Grass, A. M. (1975). Phlebo-rheographic technique for diagnosing deep venous thrombosis of the lower extremities. *Surg. Gynecol. Obstet.*, **141**, 331

18. Dahn, I. and Ericksson, E. (1968). Plethysmographic diagnosis of deep venous thrombosis of the leg. *Acta Chir. Scand.*, **398**, 33

19. DeWeese, J. A. and Rogoff, S. M. (1963). Phlebographic patterns of acute deep leg thrombosis. *Surgery*, **53**, 99

20. Dmochowski, J. R., Adams, D. F. and Couch, N. P. (1972). Impedance measurement in the diagnosis of deep venous thrombosis. *Arch. Surg.*, **104**, 170

21. Dugan, M. A., Kozar, J. J., Gause, G. and Charles, W. D. (1973). Localization of deep vein thrombosis using radioactive streptokinase. *J. Nucl. Med.*, **14**, 233

22. Evans, D. S. (1971). The early diagnosis of thromboembolism by ultrasound. *Ann. R. Coll. Surg. Engl.*, **49**, 225

23. Flanc, C., Kakkar, V. V. and Clarke, M. B. (1968). The detection of venous thrombosis of the legs using ^{125}I-labelled fibrinogen. *Br. J. Surg.*, **55**, 472

24. Flannigan, D. P., Goodreau, J. J., Burnham, S. J., Bergan, J. J., and Yao, J. S. T. (1978). Vascular-laboratory diagnosis of clinically suspected acute deep-vein thrombosis. *Lancet*, **2**, 331

25. Gallus, A. S. (1975). ^{125}I-fibrinogen leg scanning. In *Prophylactic Therapy for Deep Venous Thrombosis and Pulmonary Embolism. National Institute of Health DHEW* Publication No. 76–866, p. 77

26. Gallus, A. S., Hirsh, J., Hull, R. and van Aken, W. G. (1976). Diagnosis of venous thromboembolism. *Semin. Thromb. Hemostas.*, **2**, 203

27. Gazzaniga, A. B., Pacela, A. F., Bartlett, R. H. and Geraghty, T. R. (1972). Bilateral impedance rheography in the diagnosis of deep venous thrombosis of the legs. *Arch. Surg.*, **104**, 515

28. Grintzig, A., Bolinger, A. and Zehender, O. (1971). Moeglickeiten und grenzen der qualitativen venen-diagnostik mit Doppler ultraschall (Ergebnisse einer blind Studie). *Klin. Wochenschr.*, **49**, 245

29. Gruber, U. F. (1977). Klinische diagnostik thromboembolischer komplicationen, radiofibrinogentest, thermographie dopplersonde. *Langenbecks. Arch. Chir.*, **345**, 331

30. Harris, W.H., Athanasoulis, C., Waltman, A. C. and Salzman, E. W. (1976).

Cuff impedance phlebography and ^{125}I-fibrinogen scanning versus roentgenographic phlebography for diagnosis of thrombophlebitis following hip surgery. *J. Bone Jt. Surg.*, **58A**, 939

31. Hartsuck, J. M. and Greenfield, L. J. (1973). Postoperative thromboembolism: a clinical study with ^{125}I-fibrinogen and pulmonary scanning. *Arch. Surg.*, **107**, 733

32. Highman, J. H., O'Sullivan, E. and Thomas, E. (1973). Isotope venography. *Br. J. Surg.*, **60**, 62

33. Hirsh, J. and Hull, R. (1978). Comparative value of tests for the diagnosis of venous thrombosis. *World J. Surg.*, **2**, 27

34. Holmes, M. C. G. (1973). Deep venous thrombosis of the lower limbs diagnosed by ultrasound. *Med. J. Aust.*, **1**, 427

35. Hume, M., Kuriakose, T. X., Jamieson, J. and Turner, R. H. (1975). Extent of leg vein thrombosis determined by impedance and ^{125}I-fibrinogen. *Am. J. Surg.*, **129**, 455

36. Johnson, W. C., Patten, D. A., Widrich, W. C. and Nabseth, D. C. (1974). Technetium 99m isotope venography. *Am. J. Surg.*, **127**, 424

37. Johnston, K. W. and Kakkar, V. V. (1974). Plethysmographic diagnosis of deep vein thrombosis. *Surg. Gynecol. Obstet.*, **139**, 41

38. Kakkar, V. V. and Flanc, C. (1968). Role of phlebography in deep vein thrombosis. *Br. J. Surg.*, **55**, 384

39. Kakkar, V. V., Nicolaides, A. N., Renney, J. T. G., Friend, J. R., and Clarke, M. B. (1972). ^{125}I-labelled fibrinogen test adapted for routine screening for deep vein thrombosis. *Lancet*, **1**, 540

40. Kakkar, V. V. (1975). Deep vein thrombosis: detection and prevention. *Circulation*, **51**, 8

41. Kerrigan, G. N., Buchanan, M. R., Cade, J. F., Regoeczi, E. and Hirsh, J. (1974). Investigation of the mechanism of false-positive ^{125}I-labelled fibrinogen scans. *Br. J. Haematol.*, **26**, 469

42. Lahnborg, G., Bergstrom, K., Friman, L. and Lagergren, H. (1974). Effect of low-dose heparin on incidence of postoperative embolism detected by photo-scanning. *Lancet*, **1**, 329

43. Lambie, J. M., Mahaffy, R. G., Barber, D. C., Karmody, A. M., Scott, M. M. and Matheson, N. A. (1970). Diagnostic accuracy in venous thrombosis. *Br. Med. J.*, **2**, 142

44. Mavor, T. E., Mahaffy, R. G., Walker, M. G., Duthie, J. S., Dahll, D. P., Gaddi, J. and Reid, G. F. (1972). Peripheral venous scanning with ^{125}I-tagged fibrinogen. *Lancet*, **1**, 661

45. McDonald, G. B., Hamilton, G. W., Barnes, R. W., Rudda, T. G., Strandness, D. E. Jr. and Nelp, W. B. (1973). Radionuclide venography. *J. Nucl. Med.*, **14**, 528

46. McFarlane, A. S. (1956). Labelling of plasma proteins with radioactive iodine. *Biochem. J.*, **62**, 135

47. Millar, W. T. and Smith, J. F. B. (1974). Localization of deep venous thrombosis using technetium 99m–labelled urokinase. *Lancet*, **2**, 695

48. Milne, R. M., Griffiths, J. M. T., Gunn, A. A. and Ruckley, C. V. (1971). Postoperative deep vein thrombosis, a comparison of diagnostic techniques. *Lancet*, **2**, 445

49. Nanson, E. M., Palko, P. D., Dick, A. A. and Fedorick, S. O. (1965). Early detection of deep venous thrombosis of the legs using I^{131}-tagged human fibrinogen, a clinical study. *Ann. Surg.*, **162**, 445

50. Negus, D., Pinto, D. J., LeQuesne, L. P., Brown, N. and Chapman, M. (1968). ^{125}I-labelled fibrinogen in the diagnosis of deep-vein thrombosis and its correlation with phlebography. *Br. J. Surg.*, **55**, 835

51. Neidhart, P., Hofer, B., Duckert, F. and Fridrich, R. (1974). Die Diagnostische verwendung von I^{131}-Urokinase. *Schweiz. Med. Wochenschr.*, **104**, 141

52. Nicolaides, A. N., Kakkar, V. V., Field, E. S. and Renney, J. T. G. (1971). The origin of deep vein thrombosis, a venographic study. *Br. J. Radiol.*, **44**, 653

53. Partch, H., Lofferer, O. and Motbeck, A. (1974). Diagnosis of established deep vein thrombosis in the leg using ^{131}I-fibrinogen. *Angiology*, **25**, 719

54. Rabinov, K. and Paulin, S. (1972). Roentgen diagnosis of venous thrombosis in the leg. *Arch. Surg.*, **104**, 134

55. Rosenthall, L. (1971). Combined inferior vena cavography, iliac venography and lung imaging with ^{99m}Tc albumin aggregates. *Radiology*, **98**, 623

56. Sasahara, A. A. (1975). The diagnosis of pulmonary embolism, current status. In *National Institute of Health DHEW* Publication No. 76–866, p. 114

57. Shoop, J. D. (1974). Why do a lung scan? *J. Am Med. Assoc.*, **229**, 567

58. Sigel, B., Felix, R., Popky, G. L. and Ipsen, G. (1972). Diagnosis of lower limb venous thrombosis by Doppler ultrasonic technique. *Arch. Surg.*, **104**, 174

59. Simon, S. A. and Krakenbuhl, B. (1977). Venous stop-flow pressure: a simple and non-invasive technique for diagnosing deep vein thrombosis. *Lancet*, **2**, 1008

60. Steer, M. L., Spotnitz, A. J., Cohen, S. I., Paulin, E. and Salzman, E. W. (1973). Limitations of impedance phlebography for diagnosis of venous thrombosis. *Arch. Surg.*, **106**, 44

61. Strandness, D. E. Jr., Schultz, R. D., Sumner, D. S. and Rushmer, R. F. (1967). Ultrasonic flow detection, a useful technique in the evaluation of peripheral vascular disease. *Am. J. Surg.*, **113**, 311

62. Strandness, D. E. Jr. (1975). Ultrasound and plethysmography in the diagnosis of acute venous thrombosis. In *National Institute of Health DHEW* Publication No. 76–866, p. 100

63. Walsh, J. J., Bonnar, J. and Wright, F. W. (1974). A study of pulmonary embolism and deep vein thrombosis after major gynaecological surgery using labelled fibrinogen, phlebography and lung scanning. *J. Obstet. Gynaecol. Br. Commonw.*, **81**, 311

64. Wheeler, H. B., Pearson, D., O'Connell, D. and Mullick, S. C. (1974). Impedance phlebography, technique interpretation and results. *Arch. Surg.*, **104**, 164

65. Wheeler, H. B., O'Donnell, J. A., Anderson, F. A., Penney, B. C., Peura, R. A. and Benedict, A. A. (1975). Bedside screening for venous thrombosis using impedance phlebography. *Angiology*, **26**, 199

66. Williams, O., Lyall, J., Vernon, M. and Croft, D. N. (1974). Ventilation-perfusion lung scanning for pulmonary emboli. *Br. Med. J.*, **1**, 600

67. Wray, R., Rimmer, D., Denham, M. and Raftery, E. B. (1974). A correlative

REFERENCES

isotopic and histological study of soleal vein thrombosis. *J. Clin. Pathol.*, **27**, 813

68. Yao, J. S. T., Gourmos, C. and Hobbs, J. T. (1972). Detection of proximal vein thrombosis by Doppler ultrasound flow-detection method. *Lancet*, **1**, 1

10

Prevention of Thromboembolism in the Non-surgical Patient

As stated earlier, pulmonary embolism is becoming a leading cause of death. It is essentially a hospital-based patient problem[8,10], being not only a postoperative phenomenon, but a common cause of death in a variety of other illnesses for which patients are hospitalized. It is extremely difficult to determine how many deaths are attributable to this problem, as most recorded death certificates are very unreliable, especially where autopsies are not performed. Usually, when sudden death occurs, especially in the hospitalized patient who has not been autopsied, it is listed as a cardiac death when in reality it may be caused by a pulmonary embolism. When an autopsy is performed much also depends on the pathologist and his thoroughness in searching for possible emboli, either at the autopsy table or later upon microscopic examination of lung sections. The usually quoted estimate of the number of deaths by pulmonary embolism in the United States is 47 000 annually[7], a figure based on the rate noted at autopsy; however, the reported incidence varies widely from 6 to 64%. The author[19] has noted a postoperative incidence at autopsy of 61%. Thromboemboli, however, vary greatly in size, and often they may not be the sole cause of death, but are noted in association with other debilitating illnesses. Many patients may survive an episode of pulmonary embolism, and these together with the fatal cases have been roughly estimated to number well over 200 000 in the United States annually[8,10,11]. Pulmonary embolism occurs most often in the elderly, immobilized individuals, and is the most frequent complication of the patient who survives a myocardial infarction[6,12,13,22,23]. In this situation it is often mistaken for a second myocardial infarction – the two may be difficult to differentiate clinically. The reported incidence in these cases ranges from 25 to 35%. It is a frequent cause of death in patients with congestive heart failure, infections such as septicaemia, pneumonia and bacterial endocarditis[5,16,17,21]; it is very common in malignancies, often causing a premature death. It occurs with some frequency in the post-partum period and with women on the Pill.

The use of anticoagulants for the prevention of thromboembolism in patients with acute myocardial infarctions has been in use for some time now. More clinical trials have been reported for this condition than for any other medical problem. Yet despite the endorsement of the American Heart Association in 1968 for the use of anticoagulation in acute myocardial infarctions, there is still no general acceptance of this recommendation. The excellent review by Chalmers et al.[6] of 32 trials with the use of coumarin/indandione or heparin or both indicated that anticoagulation for these patients does prevent a significant number of fatal thromboembolisms. They report, however, a significant risk of haemorrhage with this therapy which may account for the reluctant acceptance of this form of prevention, although the studies used exclusively intravenous heparin. For the oral anticoagulants, failures and haemorrhages may be explained by the difficulties at controlling prothrombin times and the effect of other drugs which either enhance or interfere with the action of these anticoagulants. The authors conclude that 'The popularity of low-dose heparin in the prevention of preoperative and postoperative thromboembolic phenomena makes these studies of higher doses of anticoagulants obsolete'.

The author's experience using the (small dose) subcutaneous heparin sodium schedule appears to be successful in preventing fatal thromboembolism. The study was performed without the use of controls as suggested by Chalmers et al.[6] because it was deemed unethical to do so in view of the excellent results with patients having major operations.

The author's (small dose) subcutaneous heparin regime in use for acute myocardial infarction and for the hospitalized, often critically ill patient is basically the same as that employed for the surgical patient. Following the determination of the coagulation time with the modified Dale and Laidlaw coagulometer and taking into account the weight of the patient, the dose (usually 2500 – 3500 units of aqueous heparin sodium) is administered subcutaneously every 6 hours to maintain normocoagulation levels. Patients of more than 90 kg usually have a dose of 5000 units of heparin every 6 hours. Daily coagulation times determined before the next 6-hourly administration of heparin decide whether heparin dosage is increased or decreased by 1000 units to maintain normocoagulation. The results to date indicate that the author's (small dose) regime has been successful in preventing thromboembolism and in avoiding the discouraging haemorrhages which have plagued the above-mentioned studies reviewed by Chalmers et al.[6]. In addition, it appears that the author's (small dose) regime has been successful in avoiding the mural and atrial thromboses which often complicate acute myocardial infarctions. Additional confirmation of these observations are desirable.

It has been suggested that there may come a time when all hospitalized patients with their limited activity of confinement and/or immobilization may receive small subcutaneous injections of heparin as protection against deep vein thrombosis and pulmonary thromboembolism, just as it is routine for patients to have blood counts, urine analyses and minimal blood chemical analyses as a requirement on admission to the hospital.

As for other medication in the prevention of deep vein thrombosis and pulmonary embolism in the non-operative hospitalized patient, there is little evidence as to their efficacy. These substances include aspirin, dipyridamole, hydrochloroquine and flurbiprofen. The recent report of the efficacy of sulphinpyrazone[2] in the prevention of recurrent myocardial infarction in a non-hospital population still remains to be carefully evaluated. Also, in a large retrospective study by Hennekens et al.[14] aspirin failed to prevent coronary deaths in 568 men; this too requires further confirmation.

References

1. Alpert, J. S., Smith, R., Carlson, J., Ockene, I. S., Dexter, I. and Dalen, J. E. (1976). Mortality in patients treated for pulmonary embolism. *J. Am. Med. Assoc.*, **236**, 1477
2. Anturane Reinfarction Trial Research Group (1978). *N. Engl. J. Med.*, **298**, 289
3. Brown, M. and Glassenberg, M. (1973). Mortality factors in patients with acute stroke. *J. Am. Med. Assoc.*, **234**, 1493
4. Burkitt, D. P. (1972). Varicose veins, deep vein thrombosis and haemor- rhoids, epidemiology and suggested aetiology. *Br. Med. J.*, **2**, 556
5. Carlotti, J., Hardy, J. B. Jr., Linton, R. R. and White, P. D. (1947). Pul- monary embolism in medical patients. *Am. Heart J.*, **33**, 737
6. Chalmers, T. C. Matta, R. J., Smith, H. Jr. and Kunzler, H. J. (1977). Evidence favoring the use of anticoagulants in the hospital phase of acute myocardial infarction. *N. Engl. J. Med.*, **297**, 1091
7. Coon, W. W. (1977). Epidemiology of venous thromboembolism. *Arch. Surg.*, **186**, 149
8. Dalen, J. E. and Alpert, J. S. (1975). Natural history of pulmonary embolism. *Prog. Cardiovasc. Dis.*, **17**, 258
9. Ebert, R. V. (1973). Anticoagulants in acute myocardial infarction, results of a cooperative clinical trial. *J. Am. Med. Assoc.*, **225**, 724
10. Engelberg, H. (1975). The clinical use of heparin. *Curr. Ther. Res.*, **18**, 34
11. Freiman, D. G., Suyemoto, J. and Wessler, S. (1966). Frequency of pulmon- ary thromboembolism in man. *N. Engl. J. Med.*, **272**, 1278
12. Handley, A. J., Emerson, P. A. and Fleming, P. R. (1972). Heparin in the prevention of deep vein thrombosis after myocardial infarction. *Br. Med. J.*, **3**, 436
13. Hayes, M. J., Morris, G. K. and Hampton, J. R. (1976). Lack of effect of bed rest and cigarette smoking on development of deep vein thrombosis after myocardial infarction. *Br. Heart J.*, **38**, 981
14. Hennekens, C. H., Karlson, L. K. and Rosner, B. (1978). A case-control study of regular aspirin use in coronary deaths. *Circulation*, **58**, 35

15. Marks, P. and Emerson, P. A. (1974). Increased incidence of deep vein thrombosis after myocardial infarction in non-smokers. *Br. Med. J.*, **3**, 232
16. Neuhaus, A., Bentz, R. R. and Weg, J. G. (1978). Pulmonary embolism in respiration failure. *Chest*, **73**, 4
17. Peck, B., Hoffman, G. S. and Franck, W. A. (1978). Thrombophlebitis in systemic lupus erythematosus. *J. Am. Med. Assoc.*, **240**, 1728
18. Rogers, P. H. and Sherry, S. (1976). Current status of antithrombotic therapy in cardiovascular disease. *Prog. Cardiovasc. Dis.*, **19**, 236
19. Sharnoff, J. G. (1966). Post mortem findings in 25 cases of sudden heart arrest in the perioperative period. *Lancet*, **2**, 876
20. Sion, A. and Lopez-Magano, V. (1978). Incidence of pulmonary embolism. *Respiration*, **35**, 181
21. Warlow, C. (1978). Venous thromboembolism after stroke. *Am. Heart J.*, **96**, 283
22. Warlow, C., Beattie, A. G., Terry, G., Osbon, D., Kenmure, A. C. F. and Douglas, A. S. (1973). A double-blind trial of low doses of heparin in the prevention of deep vein thrombosis after myocardial infarction. *Lancet*, **2**, 934
23. Wolf, R., Beck, O. A. and Hochrein, H. (1974). Der Einfluss von Heparin auf die Haufigkeit von Rythmusstorungen beim akuten Myokardinfarct. *Deutsch Med. Wochenschr.*, **99**, 1549

11

Monitoring Heparin Prophylaxis

The monitoring of heparin prophylaxis has long been a problem. As a result, many tests have been devised but have proved unsatisfactory for one reason or another. It was shortly before the discovery of heparin by McLean in 1916 that the Lee–White coagulation time test (1913) for blood was introduced and later used to determine the effect of heparin on coagulation. In general blood coagulation time has for many years been relied upon as the best method available. The test is performed by drawing 3 ml of venous blood in a dry glass syringe. With the needle removed, 1 ml of blood is delivered into three test tubes of standard size, 13×100 mm. A stopwatch is started when the blood is drawn into the syringe. The tubes are placed in a water bath at 37 °C and after 2 minutes tilted every 30 seconds. When clotting is noted in each tube the times are recorded and their average is reported as the coagulation time; the normal range is 5–10 minutes. The test is not precise chiefly because of the difficulty in determining the end-point and is therefore less than satisfactory. An equally unsatisfactory and little used test is the capillary tube test where fingertip blood is allowed to fill capillary glass tubes of 1 mm diameter and 5 cm length; a stopwatch is started and the tubes are broken every 30 seconds until a fibrin thread is seen between the broken ends. The normal range is 3–5 minutes.

Other tests worthy of mention recommended for the monitoring of heparin administration are the heparin tolerance test described by deTakats[10,11], the heparin assay by Denson and Bonnar[9], the thrombin time by Yin, Wessler and Butler[37], the partial thromboplastin time (PTT) and the activated partial thromboplastin time (APTT). The techniques of performing these tests are varied and involved and may be found in the cited references[17,18,29–31,35]. The value of the heparin tolerance test is questionable, as it has an extremely wide normal range and is not practical in a large series of patients. The Denson and Bonnar heparin assay is complex, not a bedside procedure, and is impractical for a large series of patients. The thrombin time test described by Yin, Wessler and Butler[37], the partial thromboplastin time and the activated partial thromboplastin time are all laboratory procedures which tend to be insensitive[2,3,5] and variable[21] chiefly due to the unrealiability of the thromboplastin[24] used. The APTT has gained greater favour and usage chiefly because of the lack of a better test. It consists of recalcifying plasma in the presence of a standardized amount of platelet reagent and a plasma activator. It is a modification of the PTT wherein a reagent is added capable of fully activating factors XI and XII prior to recalcification. It is considered to be more sensitive than the PTT and deemed useful as a screening test only. It has been used to monitor heparin, often with unsatisfactory results[21]. The latter is ascribed to commonly used medication which can reduce or increase clotting times. For valid results extreme care must be taken when performing the test and in the interpretion of the results; the normal range is 35–50 seconds. Here again it is not practical to perform a large number of daily determinations, nor is it suitable for rapid determination at the bedside. Although it is preferred by most clinicians, it is not of much use in making rapid decisions as to heparin dosage at the bedside. The same may be said of the methods described by Yin, and Denson and Bonnar; the latter method is based on the inactivation of factor Xa. Teien and Lie[32], in evaluating five clotting methods including several mentioned above, found that the polybrene titration method is the most reliable although it is too cumbersome for practical use. This method also is of little use in making rapid decisions as to dosage at the patient's bedside.

An extremely simple, reproducible bedside whole blood clotting method for monitoring heparin administration is the author's modified Dale and Laidlaw coagulometer[26]*. This has proved highly effective in avoiding the problems encountered in the fixed (low dose) regime, namely the serious haemorrhages and wound haematomas. It has been indispensible in the author's variable (small dose) heparin regime and is the chief reason for the latter programme's success. The coagulometer method permits an immediate determination of the anticoagulant therapy and for the adjustment of heparin dosage if needed. It is a practical and inexpensive test that can be done on a large number of patients in a very short time; it can be learnt quickly because of its simplicity. Also, it can measure the action of the oral anticoagulants such as coumadin and warfarin long before the prothrombin time values are altered.

The test is performed with a capillary glass tube measuring 1.5 cm in length and 1.5 mm in diameter. The tube contains a stainless steel ball weighing *exactly* 0.7 mg. The weight is critical. The tube is narrowed at both ends to stop the ball falling out, and it can roll freely back and forth in the tube. The tube should be checked for this before commencing the test. The equipment required for the test consists of a water bath, which must be well lighted and maintained at 37 °C, a stopwatch and a sterile disposable lancet. The test is performed by first wiping a fingertip clean with an alcohol sponge and then allowing it to dry. The ball of the finger is pricked well with the lancet and the stopwatch is started. With the hand held in supination a drop of blood is permitted to puddle on the ball of the finger. One end of the tube is touched to the blood puddle which allows the tube to fill quickly with blood by capillary action. The tube is immediately immersed in the water with both ends sealed by holding it between the thumb and index finger. The tube is then tilted slowly from end to end so that the steel ball rolls slowly back and forth. The ball must be kept in view at all times for it will stop rolling suddenly and the endpoint may be missed. When the ball stops rolling, the sharp endpoint is

* Available from R.G. Finnie, 16 Binghill Road, West Milltimber, Aberdeen, Scotland.

reached and no attempt should be made to start the ball rolling again by shaking the tube vigorously. The time is recorded using the stopwatch.

The normal range is 1.5–2.5 minutes. Experience has shown that maintaining blood coagulation in this range with heparin will prevent thrombosis and further propagation of already existing thrombi. The sharpness of the endpoint has made this test most reliable in contrast to the Lee–White coagulation time[26]. It has accounted for the success of the author's (small dose) variable heparin programme in the prevention and treatment of thrombosis for the past 15 years, and has been the means of avoiding the serious complication of frequent haemorrhage encountered with other programmes especially the fixed (low dose) programme. As the latter does not recommend monitoring of heparin therapy this accounts for the haemorrhages and haematomas encountered with that programme, and this has caused many investigators to abandon it after short trials. Despite this, the Thrombosis Council of the American Heart Association in recommending the fixed (low dose) regime stated that 'No laboratory test (whole blood clotting time, partial thromboplastin time, thrombin time and antithrombin III assay) is necessary during therapy to determine dosage as to prevent haemorrhage. It must be clearly recognized that the low dose heparin regime may minimally increase the likelihood of such haemorrhage. . . . The low dose regimen has not proved effective in open prostatectomies or major orthopedic operations.' Also, to quote D. P. Thomas, 'this regimen (low dose heparin) is well tolerated by the patient and requires no laboratory monitoring'[34]. Barrowcliffe, Johnson and Thomas[1] quoting Brozovic and Bangham[4] state that 'the in vitro assays of heparin reveal a bewildering variety of methods, most of which measure different aspects of the clotting mechanism and are therefore not clinically useful'. There are many additional reports confirming the inefficacy of these assays, and this may account for the recommendation that the fixed (low dose) regimen does not require monitoring.

Charnley[6] was one of the first to abandon the fixed (low dose) regime for patients having hip surgery, because of several haemorrhages and fatal embolisms after using it in 47 patients. String and Barcia[28] reported a 13.7% incidence of wound haematomas using the fixed (low dose) schedule. Kakkar, Corrigan and Fossard reporting in the International Multicenter Trial had a 16.6% complication rate due to excess blood loss. Gruber *et al.*[15] reported a 14% incidence of haemorrhage and wound haematomas with two patients requiring reoperation to control bleeding. More recently, Pachter and Riles[21] in a study of 175 randomized prospective surgical patients, using the fixed (low dose) regimen in 66 patients, postoperative heparin only in one control group and no heparin in a second control group, reported a 27% incidence of haemorrhage and wound haematomas in the fixed (low dose) heparin group. Compared with this the postoperative heparin group had a 7.5% incidence of haemorrhage and the no-heparin group had a 1.4% incidence of haemorrhage and wound haematomas. They concluded, 'In treating these high risk patients with low dose heparin, however, one should be prepared to exchange a decrease in deep vein thrombosis and pulmonary emboli for a high bleeding and wound complication rate'. All of their patients were treated by the fixed (low dose) heparin regimen and not monitored. There are a number of additional reports confirming the same[15,19,28,31]. To quote deTakats[12] again,

> To avoid major bleeding which occurs in 7–8% of patients in most series, the doses represent a compromise between amounts that would offer more protection against thrombosis and those that are apt to result in haemorrhage . . . . This is the curse of the rigid schedule. Not only is there great individual variation in the response to heparin but also the magnitude and length of the operation influence the clotting fibrinolytic balance. Each patient has his or her own heparin tolerance and own fibrinolytic potential and the clotting mechanism can be monitored by simple bedside tests . . . and lately [the author] has shown that prophylactic heparin doses are practical even after treatment of hip fractures when monitored.

The above are sound observations and although the variation from patient to patient is not too great, monitoring is necessary to pick up the one individual who deviates from the norm. Monitoring with the author's modified Dale and Laidlaw coagulometer[26] has made possible the safe and simple treatment for the prevention of thromboembolism with subcutaneous 'small doses' of heparin. Eighteen years of experience in more than 6000 cases amply confirms this.

References

1. Barrowcliffe, T. W., Johnson, E. A. and Thomas, D. P. (1978). Antithrombin III and heparin. *Br. Med. Bull.*, **34**, 143
2. Basu, D., Gallus, A., Hirsh, J. and Cade, J. (1972). A prospective study of the value of monitoring heparin treatment with the activated partial thromboplastin time. *N. Engl. J. Med.*, **287**, 324
3. Bonnar, J. and Denson, K. W. E. (1973). Monitoring of heparin. *Thromb. Diath. Haemorrh.*, **30**, 471
4. Brozovic, M. and Bangham, D. R. (1975). Heparin structure, function and clinical implications. In Bradshaw, R. A. and Wessler, S. (eds.) *Advances in Experimental Medicine and Biology*, Vol. 52, pp. 163–79. (New York and London: Plenum Press)
5. Bull, M. H., Huse, W. M. and Bull, B. S. (1975). Evaluation of tests used to monitor heparin therapy during extracorporeal circulation. *Anaesthesiology*, **43**, 346
6. Charnley, J. (1972). Prophylaxis of postoperative thromboembolism. *Lancet*, **2**, 134
7. Cooke, E. D., Lloyd, M. J., Bowcock, S. A. and Pilcher, M. F. (1976). Monitoring during low-dose heparin prophylaxis. *N. Engl. J. Med.*, **294**, 1066
8. Davis, J. J. (1975). Monitoring during low dose heparin prophylaxis. *N. Engl. J. Med.*, **293**, 776
9. Denson, K. W. E. and Bonnar, J. (1973). The measurement of heparin. A method based on the potentiation of antifactor Xa. *Thromb. Diath. Haemorrh.*, **30**, 471
10. deTakats, G. (1943). Heparin tolerance, a test of the clotting mechanism. *Surg. Gynecol. Obstet.*, **77**, 31
11. deTakats, G. (1971). Heparin tolerance revisited. *Surgery*, **70**, 318
12. deTakats, G. (1977). Small-dose prophylactic heparin, does it prevent venous thrombosis? *Mod. Med.*, 38
13. Genton, E. (1974). Guidelines for heparin therapy. *Ann. Intern. Med.*, **89**, 77
14. Gormsen, J. and Haxholdt, B. Fl. (1960). The heparin tolerance test and thromboembolic incidence in surgery. *Acta Chir. Scand.*, **120**, 121

15. Gruber, V. F., Duckert, F., Fridrich, R., Torhorst, J. and Rem, J. (1977). Prevention of postoperative thromboembolism by dextran 40, low doses of heparin and xantinol nicotinate. *Lancet*, **1**, 207

16. Kazmier, F. J. (1976). A significant interaction between metronidazole and warfarin. *Mayo Clin. Proc.*, **5**, 782

17. Koepke, J. A. (1975). The partial thromboplastin time in the C. A. P. survey program. *Am. J. Clin. Pathol.*, **63**, 990

18. Makarg, A. L. and Waterbury, V. (1977). The activated partial thromboplastin time as a monitor of heparin: a warning. *Johns Hopkins Med. J.*, **140**, 311

19. Mant, M. J., O'Brien, B. D., Thong, K. L., Hammond, G. W., Birtwhistle, R. V. and Grace, M. G. (1977). Hemorrhagic complications of heparin therapy. *Lancet*, **1**, 1133

20. Multicentre Trial (1975). Prevention of fatal postoperative pulmonary embolism by low doses of heparin. *Lancet*, **2**, 45

21. Pachter, H. L. and Riles, T. S. (1977). Bleeding and wound complications in the surgical patient, a prospective randomized study. *Ann. Surg.*, **186**, 669

22. Penner, J. A. (1974). Experience with a thrombin clotting time assay for measuring heparin activity. *Am. J. Clin. Pathol.*, **61**, 645

23. Poller, L., Thomson, J. H. and Yee, K. F. (1977). Stability studies on lyophilized reference thromboplastins for standardization of prothrombin times. *Lancet*, **2**, 1019

24. Prevention of venous thromboembolism in surgical patients by low dose heparin. (1977). *Circulation*, **55**, 423A

25. Shapiro, G. A., Huntzinger, S. W. and Wilson, J. E. (1977). Variation among commercial activated partial thromboplastin time reagents in response to heparin. *Am. J. Clin. Pathol.*, **67**, 477

26. Sharnoff, J. G. (1963). An evaluation of the Dale and Laidlaw coagulometer in heparin control of thromboembolism. *NY State Assoc. Pub. Hlth. Lab.*, **43**, 10

27. Sharnoff, J. G. (1977). Low-dose or small-dose heparin. *Lancet*, **2**, 1087

28. String, S. T. and Barcia, P. J. (1975). Complications of small dose prophylactic heparinization. *Am. J. Surg.*, **130**, 570

29. Sherry, S. (1971). Thrombosis prevention. *N. Engl. J. Med.*, **284**, 1324

30. Soloway, H. B., Cornett, B. M. and Grayson, J. W. (1972). Comparison of various activated partial thrombo-reagents in the laboratory control of heparin therapy. *Am. J. Clin. Pathol.*, **39**, 587

31. Taberner, D. A., Poller, L., Burslem, R. W. and Jones, J. B. (1978). Oral anticoagulants controlled by the British comparative thromboplastin versus low-dose heparin in prophylaxis of deep vein thrombosis. *Br. Med. J.*, **1**, 272

32. Teien, A. N. and Lie, M. (1975). Heparin assay in plasma. A comparison of five clotting methods. *Thromb. Res.*, **7**, 777

33. Teien, A. N., Lie, M. and Abildgard, U. (1976). Assay of heparin in plasma using a chromagenic substance for activated factor X. *Thromb. Res.*, **8**, 413

34. Thomas, D. P. (1977). Low-dose heparin. *Lancet*, **2**, 1181

35. Triplett, D. A., Harms, G. J. and Koepke, J. A. (1978). The effect of heparin in activated partial thromboplastin times. *Am. J. Clin. Pathol.*, **70**, 556

REFERENCES

36. Wessler, S. and Gitel, S. (1976). Control of heparin therapy. *Prog. Hemostas. Thromb.*, **3**, 311
37. Yin, E. T., Wessler, S. and Butler, J. V. (1973). Plasma heparin, a unique practical submicrogram-sensitive assay. *J. Lab. Clin. Med.*, **8**, 298

12
Therapy of Deep Vein Thrombosis and Thromboembolism

In the presence of deep vein thrombosis and thromboembolism, anticoagulant therapy remains the treatment of choice against which all other means of therapy must be measured. Despite this there are available many varieties of treatment of thrombosis and embolism reflecting the unsatisfactory results that have been obtained from the use of oral anticoagulants. Before the introduction of subcutaneous heparin, oral anticoagulants[15] and intravenous heparin[4] remained the best methods at hand to treat thrombosis. But the high incidence of haemorrhage and the failure of treatment has caused considerable disenchantment[29].

Before discussing the subcutaneous heparin therapeutic approach[11], a review of the other means of therapy will be presented. Recent developments have made the use of leg elevation and ace bandaging obsolete, so it is more pertinent to review the status of such means of therapy as streptokinase, urokinase, snake venoms, surgical venous interruption and pulmonary embolectomy.

There appears to be no question that streptokinase is an effective thrombolytic agent[3,9,16,35]. It is a soluble product of the metabolism of *Streptococcus pyogenes*. Fresh fibrin clots are sensitive to streptokinase, whereas clots older than 24 hours are less sensitive. Because it is antigenic to man it may produce antibodies, and earlier infections with *Streptococci* may produce resistance to its action and create dosage problems. It can also cause pyrexia, dyspnoea and tachycardia, and acts by transforming plasminogen to plasmin, the active fibrinolytic enzyme. It may be made cheaply in large quantities. Because of the problems with its use and the difficulty of obtaining consistent laboratory determination of fibrinogen and its split products, it has not attained common use, and in venous thrombosis and pulmonary thromboembolism it has now been superseded by the use of adequate doses of heparin sodium.

Urokinase[17,20,21,25,26], another thrombolytic agent with the same action as streptokinase, is derived from human urine. As such it takes large quantities of human urine for its production, making it very expensive medication, although now it is prepared from cultures of renal tissues. It has been proved an effective thrombolytic agent as a direct plasminogen activator but it may produce a prolonged state of plasminaemia and therefore uncontrollable haemorrhages. This may in part be due to the inability of laboratory tests such as thrombin time and determination of fibrinogen and split products to assess its action and dosage. It too, like streptokinase, is effective when fibrin is fresh. As with streptokinase, it has not been commercially available until recently and heparin has also superseded it as a therapeutic agent for thrombosis. It may also be said that in the event of thromboembolism, if the patient survives long enough to establish the diagnosis, then it may be too late to initiate thrombolytic therapy and the patient may survive without therapy anyway.

The snake venoms Arvin and reptilase[6,19] have also been used as therapy in thromboembolism. Arvin is derived from the Malayan pit viper *Ancistrodon rhodostoma*. In 1963 Reid *et al.*[46] observed the general haemorrhagic syndrome found in victims of bites by the viper. Arvin is the name given to the purified fraction of the crude venom, and reptilase is derived from the South American pit viper *Bothrops atrox*. The action of both is similar, functioning as a proteolytic enzyme producing fibrinolysis. Most studies to date indicate that these substances have an anticoagulant effect. The most common and serious complication of this form of therapy is bleeding. As a result, snake venom therapy is contraindicated after recent surgery, in pregnancy, and in patients with thrombocytopenia, pulmonary embolism and circulatory deficiencies. In con-

119

clusion, it may be said that no final decision can be made on the value of these snake venoms in the therapy of venous thrombosis and pulmonary thromboembolism. Again heparin therapy should be the treatment of choice.

The most commonly used surgical approach to the treatment of pulmonary thromboembolism is venous interruption. The methods used have been femoral vein ligation, inferior vena cava ligation, inferior vena cava plication and the intraluminal techniques. Embolectomy is the least common surgical method employed, although it was the earliest method tried. Femoral vein ligation has been abandoned in favour of inferior vena cava interruption due to the poor results experienced in the former, such as high incidence of operative mortality, recurrent phlebothrombosis and fatal embolism.

Inferior vena cava ligation[5,13,28,37,40-42] became popular 25 years ago. Ligation is usually carried out just below the renal vein. Although results were somewhat better than with femoral vein ligation the postoperative mortality rate and sequelae[11,43,44] have limited its use. First reported by Bottini in 1893 it had little use until suggested by Homans in 1944[27] and in 1945 by O'Neil[42] when it became more commonly used in the prevention of recurrent thromboembolism. More recently inferior vena cava plication has become preferable; here suturing or stapling of the inferior vena cava has been partly replaced by the use of filters or clips[24]. Among the latter, the DeWeese filter[14], the suturing or stapling of the vena cava[5], the Moretz[33], Miles, and Adams–DeWeese clips[1] can be mentioned. Each have their own advocates. The evidence to date is that each method can reduce the incidence of recurrent pulmonary embolism but cannot completely eliminate it. There are well documented reports that, depending on the site of caval interruption or plication, the collateral circulation, such as the spermatic or ovarian veins and the epigastric veins, may give rise to emboli. Also, it is known that thrombosis above the site of caval interruption has also caused emboli and deaths. In addition embolism may originate from the right heart or upper extremities. The results reported with the use of plication have been superior to that of ligation, but as mentioned above, phlebothrombosis and fat emboli are still reported though reduced in number. Thus the procedure is resorted to only when anticoagulation has failed. The DeWeese filter and the clips devised by Adams, Miles, and Moretz have the rationale of not entirely occluding blood flow with the leg oedema and skin ulcerations that result with ligation. The operative results appear to be slightly better than ligation yet the same complications such as proximal thrombosis and fatal thromboembolism still occur with some frequency. It has also been noted that all these methods often lead to complete thrombosis at the site of plication and result in the equivalent of ligation[12].

In very recent years a number of intraluminal techniques[24,32,36] have been introduced in an effort to improve on the operative mortality rate encountered with the inferior vena cava plication methods. These include the Mobin-Uddin umbrella, the Eichelter sieve and the Pate clip[5] all into a peripheral vein and eventually lodge in the inferior vena cava. Here a simple operation is required. They have the disadvantage of possibly dislodging a thrombus proximal to the point of installation, namely the iliac vein or the inferior vena cava.

Although the introduction of these devices performed under local anaesthesia is simple and controlled by fluoroscopy a significant number of patients have had difficulties with these procedures. The problems have been placement of the device in the major veins through the neck approach and misplacement in the renal or iliac veins. Here also thrombi have been reported dislodged as emboli and the device dislodged as an embolus. It has also been reported that the mortality rate with the Mobin-Uddin umbrella[36] is not improved over that of the plication methods. However, these methods of caval interruption are steadily decreasing in favour of management with anticoagulants, especially with the use of subcutaneous heparin sodium therapy. The latter has proved highly effective in treating deep vein thrombosis and preventing recurrent thromboembolism. Two additional intraluminal techniques have been tried to a limited extent – the Hunter[28] and Moser[39] balloon catheters introduced through the jugular vein.

The oldest surgical approach, pulmonary embolectomy, was first performed by Trendelenburg in 1908, who proposed that when pulmonary embolism was suspected, the pulmonary artery should be opened and the embolus removed[31]. More patients died in such attempts than survived and the method was virtually abandoned until recently[34,35] newer techniques, including the use of extracorporeal circulation and angiography performed for diagnostic confirmation[48], were introduced. These are now essential requirements before surgical intervention is attempted. However, to complete the study and prepare the patient requires time; in most instances death occurs too rapidly to allow the time required for embolectomy.

Therefore, the standard against which all of the above therapeutic means must be measured is anticoagulation with heparin therapy as the means in most common use. Until recently intravenous heparin therapy was the method most often employed. The usual dosage recommended was sufficient heparin injected every four hours to attain Lee–White coagulation to two to three times normal values. Unfortunately the haemorrhages and fatalities that resulted have caused great discouragement with its use[29].

At present the most satisfactory approach in the author's extensive experience[47] seems to be the subcutaneous sodium heparin method. Although there appears to be little evidence that heparin can dissolve already present thrombi or emboli, the rapid response to this form of therapy is most striking. This may well be due to the fact that heparin in small doses given subcutaneously to maintain normocoagulable levels prevents further propagation of the thrombus and hastens recanalization of the already present thrombus.

Our results with the (small dose) heparin sodium regime controlled by the author's modified Dale and Laidlaw coagulometer has been most satisfactory with clinical improvement noticeable within 24–48 hours following the institution of therapy. As described earlier the routine employed has been the following. After clinical confirmation or by venography of the presence of a deep vein thrombosis a baseline coagulation time with the coagulometer must first be obtained and then 2500–5000 units of sodium heparin (depending on body weight) must be administered every 6 hours with daily determinations of coagulation times. Heparin dosage is adjusted by increasing or decreasing dosage by 1000 units if necessary until the patient is fully reactivated or discharged from the hospital. But for the operative patient alone the need for this form of therapy may also be greatly reduced if the preoperative prophylaxis approach is universally adopted (this has been described earlier). It is not necessary to either increase the subcutaneous heparin dose or use large doses of intravenous heparin as suggested by Wessler[51] and others[30,49]. The same may be said of the use of continuous intravenous infusion as suggested by Thomas[50].

References

1. Adams, J. T. and DeWeese, J. A. (1966). Partial interruption of inferior vena cava with new plastic clip. *Surg. Gynecol. Obstet.*, **133**, 1087
2. Allison, P. R., Dunnill, N. S. and Marshall, R. (1960). Pulmonary embolism. *Thorax*, **15**, 273
3. Arneson, H., Heilo, A., Jakobsen, E., Ly, B. and Skaga, E. (1978). A prospective study of streptokinase and heparin in the treatment of deep vein thrombosis. *Acta Med. Scand.*, **203**, 457
4. Barritt, D. W. and Jordan, S. C. (1960). Anticoagulant drugs in the treatment of pulmonary embolism, a controlled trial. *Lancet*, **1**, 1309
5. Bernstein, E. F. (1978). The role of operative inferior vena caval interruption in the management of venous thromboembolism. *World. J. Surg.*, **2**, 61
6. Blomback, M., Egberg, N., Grude, E., Johansson, S. A., Johansson, H., Nilson, S. E. G. and Blomback, B. (1971). Treatment of thrombotic disorders with reptilase. *Thromb. Diath. Haemorrh. Suppl.*, **45**, 50
7. Browse, N. L. (1978). Natural fibrinolysis. *Am. Heart J.*, **95**, 417
8. Browse, N. L. (1974). Current thoughts on venous thromboembolism. *Surg. Clin. N. Am.*, **54**, 229
9. Chesterman, C. N. (1973). Results of streptokinase therapy in pulmonary embolism. *Postgrad. Med. J.*, **49** (Suppl.5), 78
10. Clark, W. B., MacGregor, A. B., Prescott, R. J. and Ruckley, C. V. (1974). Pneumatic compression of the calf and postoperative deep vein thrombosis. *Lancet*, **2**, 5
11. Coon, W. W. (1978). Anticoagulant therapy for venous thromboembolism. *Postgrad. Med.*, **63**, 157
12. Coupland, C. A. E. and Reeve, T. S. (1970). Recurrent pulmonary emboli following inferior vena caval ligation. *Surgery*, **67**, 639
13. Dale, W. A. (1958). Ligation of the inferior vena cava for thromboembolism. *Surgery*, **43**, 22 (Cites Bottini, 1893)
14. DeWeese, M. S. and Hunter, D. C. (1958). A vena caval filter for the prevention of pulmonary emboli. *Bull. Soc. Int. Chir.*, **17**, 17
15. Deykin, D. (1970). Warfarin therapy. *N. Engl. J. Med.*, **283**, 691

REFERENCES

16. Duckert, F., Muller, G., Nyman, D., Benz, A., Prisender, S., Madar, G., DaSilva, M. A., Widmer, L. K. and Schmitt, H. E. (1975). Treatment of deep vein thrombosis with streptokinase. *Br. Med. J.*, **1**, 479
17. Edwards, I. R., McLean, K. S. and Dow, J. D. (1973). Low-dose urokinase in major pulmonary embolism. *Lancet*, **2**, 409
18. Eichelter, P. and Schenk, W. G. Jr. (1968). Prophylaxis of pulmonary embolism. A new experimental approach with initial results. *Arch. Surg.*, **97**, 348
19. Egeberg, O., Blomback, M., Johansson, H., Abildgaard, U., Blomback, B., Diener, G., McDonagh, J., McDonagh, L., Ekestrom, S., Goransson, B., Johansson, S. A., Nilson, S. E., Nordstrom, S., Olsson, P. and Wiman, B. (1971). Clinical and experimental studies on reptilase. *Thromb. Diath. Haemorrh., Suppl.*, **47**, 370
20. Fletcher, A. P., Alkjaersig, N., Sherry, S., Genton, E., Hirsh, J. and Bachmann, F. (1965). The development of urokinase as a thrombolytic agent. Maintenance of a sustained thrombolytic state in man by its intravenous infusion. *J. Lab. Clin. Med.*, **65**, 713
21. Genton, E. and Wolf, P. S. (1968). Urokinase therapy in pulmonary thromboembolism. *Am. Heart J.*, **76**, 628
22. Gorham, L. W. (1961). A study of pulmonary embolism, Part I. *Arch. Intern. Med.*, **108**, 8
23. Gorham, L. W. (1961). A study of pulmonary embolism, Part II. *Arch. Intern. Med.*, **108**, 189
24. Greenfield, L. J. (1978). Intraluminal techniques for vena caval interruption and pulmonary embolectomy. *World J. Surg.*, **2**, 45
25. Gurevich, V. and Thomas, D. P. (1970). Streptokinase in acute pulmonary embolism, an experimental study. *J. Thorac. Cardiovasc. Surg.*, **59**, 655
26. Hirsh, J., Hale, G. S., McDonald, I. G., McCarthy, R. A. and Pitt, A. (1968). Streptokinase therapy in acute major pulmonary embolism: effectiveness and problems. *Br. Med. J.*, **4**, 729
27. Homans, J. (1944). Deep quiet venous thrombosis in the lower limb. *Surg. Gynecol. Obstet.*, **79**, 70
28. Hunter, J. A., Dye, W. S., Javid, H., Najati, N., Goldin, M. D. and Serry, C. (1977). Permanent transvenous occlusion of inferior vena cava. *Ann. Surg.*, **186**, 49
29. Jick, H., Slone, D., Borda, I. T. and Shapiro, S. (1968). Efficacy and toxicity of heparin in relation to age and sex. *N. Engl. J. Med.*, **279**, 284
30. Kakkar, V. V. and Raftery, E. B. (1970). Selection of patients with pulmonary embolism for thrombolytic therapy. *Lancet*, **2**, 237
31. Kirschner, M. (1924). Ein durch die Trendelenburgsche operation geheilte fall von emboli der arterie pulmonales. *Arch. Klin. Chir.*, **133**, 312
32. Lawrence, G. H. and Beebe, H. G. (1976). An evaluation of the Mobin-Uddin umbrella in the prevention of pulmonary thromboembolism. *Am. J. Surg.*, **132**, 204
33. Leather, R. P., Clark, W. R., Powers, S. P., Parker, F. B., Bernard, H. R. and Eckert, C. (1968). Five year experience with the Moretz clip in 62 patients. *Arch. Surg.*, **97**, 357

34. Meyerowitz, B. R. (1966). Pulmonary embolism in surgical patients: is embolectomy superior to prophylaxis? *Surgery*, **60**, 521
35. Miller, G. A. H., Hall, R. J. C. and Paneth, M. (1977). Pulmonary embolectomy, heparin and streptokinase: their place in treatment of acute massive pulmonary embolism. *Am. Heart J.*, **93**, 568
36. Mobin-Uddin, K., Uttley, J. R. and Bryant, L. R. (1975). The inferior vena cava umbrella filter. *Prog. Cardiovasc. Dis.*, **17**, 391
37. Moran, J. M., Kahn, P. C. and Callow, A. D. (1969). Partial versus complete interruption for venous thromboembolism. *Am. J. Surg.*, **117**, 471
38. Morris, G. K. and Mitchell, J. R. A. (1978). Clinical management of venous thromboembolism. *Br. Med. Bull.*, **34**, 169
39. Moser, K. M. (1977). Pulmonary embolism. *Am. Rev. Resp. Dis.*, **115**, 829
40. Mozes, M., Gobolowsky, H., Antebi, E., Tzur, N. and Penchas, S. (1966). Inferior vena cava ligation for pulmonary embolism. *Surgery*, **60**, 790
41. Ochsner, A., Ochsner, J. L. and Sanders, H. S. (1970). Prevention of pulmonary embolism by caval ligation. *Ann. Surg.*, **171**, 923
42. O'Neill, E. E. (1945). Vena caval ligation for phlebothrombosis. *N. Engl. J. Med.*, **232**, 641
43. Piccone, V. A., Vidal, E., Yarnoz, M., Glass, B. S. and LeVeen, H. H. (1970). The late results of caval ligation. *Surgery*, **68**, 980
44. Pollack, E. W., Sparks, F. C. and Barker, W. F. (1974). Inferior vena cava interruptions, indications and results with caval ligation, clips and intraluminal devices. *J. Cardiovasc. Surg.*, **15**, 629
45. Reichel, J. (1977). Pulmonary embolism. *Med. Clin. N. Am.*, **61**, 1309
46. Reid, R. A., Thean, P. C., Chan, K. E. and Baharon, A. R. (1963). Clinical effects of bites of Malayan viper (*Ancistrodon rhodostoma*). *Lancet*, **1**, 617
47. Sharnoff, J. G. Unpublished data
48. Sharp, E. H. (1962). Pulmonary embolectomy: successful removal of a massive pulmonary embolus with support of cardiopulmonary bypass, a case report. *Ann. Surg.*, **156**, 1
49. Tibbutt, D. A. and Chesterman, C. N. (1976). Pulmonary embolism: current therapeutic concepts. *Drugs*, **11**, 161
50. Thomas, D. P. (1978). Heparin in the prophylaxis and treatment of venous thromboembolism. *Semin. Hematol.*, **15**, 1
51. Wessler, S. (1976). Medical management of venous thrombosis. *Ann. Rev. Med.*, **27**, 313

13

Other Problems of Major Surgery Avoided by Heparin Prophylaxis

A number of other serious conditions which complicate major surgery can be prevented by the use of subcutaneous heparin prophylaxis. One extremely dangerous complication which has not been noted clinically by the author in more than 3000 successful cases using (small dose) heparin prophylaxis is the acute stress ulcer with exsanguinating haemorrhage and/or perforation followed by death due to peritonitis. Although as yet unconfirmed by controlled trials it has also been observed by the Mount Sinai Hospital clinicians[1]. The acute stress ulcers are commonly seen in the stomach or duodenum, and are often multiple in number causing massive intestinal haemorrhage and/or perforation. Their underlying cause has been demonstrated pathologically by Margaretten and McKay[2], and confirmed by the author at autopsy as small vessel thromboses in the submucosa of the bowel in 70% of cases. It can be assumed that these thrombi occur during surgery and are prevented by the administration of heparin sodium preoperatively.

Although studies reported by the author[4] on the incidence of cardiopulmonary arrests in the perioperative period have limited statistical evidence, it appears that this complication can also be prevented by the preoperative administration of subcutaneous heparin[5]. These studies also disclosed at autopsy that cardiopulmonary arrests were induced by pulmonary thromboembolisms, and that the size of the emboli ranged from massive to microemboli[4] – the latter often being a shower of many small emboli. In a few instances the cardiopulmonary arrests were also induced by coronary artery thromboses[4]. It also appears, from clinical evidence in the author's series of patients that the latter can be prevented by subcutaneous heparin prophylaxis. This too requires further substantiation. No other forms of arterial thromboses have been observed with this kind of prophylaxis, such as cerebral, mesenteric, coronary and renal thromboses and infarctions.

There is also evidence that the length of hospitalization is significantly shortened by heparin prophylaxis. This was observed in a review of a large series of patients having surgery for hip fracture; the heparinized patients had a shorter hospitalization by 4–5 days compared to the non-heparinized patients.

Evidence is also increasing that the preoperative prophylactic use of subcutaneous heparin may also prevent another frequent complication of major surgery, namely renal tubular necrosis. This is manifested by the infrequent observation of anuria and elevation of urea nitrogen with the use of the author's (small dose) subcutaneous heparin regime.

All these added benefits are in need of further confirmation. There is no question any longer that the subcutaneous (small dose) heparin prophylaxis regime as described here is simple to administer, entirely safe from haemorrhage, and with proper, simple bedside control it will prevent not only the above complications of major surgery but, most important, deep vein thrombosis and the possibility of thromboembolism.

References

1. Bryan-Brown, C. W. and Adler, D. C. (1974). Low-dose heparin and stress ulceration. *Lancet*, **2**, 1078
2. Margaretten, W. and McKay, D. G. (1971). Thrombotic ulcerations of the gastro-intestinal tract. *Arch. Intern. Med.*, **127**, 250
3. Ming, S. C. (1965). Hemorrhagic necrosis of the gastro-intestinal tract and its relation to cardiovascular status. *Circulation*, **32**, 332
4. Sharnoff, J. G. (1966). Post mortem findings in 25 cases of sudden heart arrest in the perioperative period. *Lancet*, **2**, 876
5. Sharnoff, J. G. (1969). Prevention of sudden cardio-pulmonary arrest in the perioperative period with prophylactic heparin. *Lancet*, **2**, 292
6. Sharnoff, J. G. and DeBlasio, G. (1970). Some implications in the successful prophylaxis of sudden cardio-pulmonary arrest by thrombosis and embolism. *Am. Heart J.*, **80**, 848

Index